Ketogenic Vegetarian & Keto Bread – 2 books in 1

Delicious Recipes for Healthy Lifestyle and Weight Loss

Written By

Allyson C. Naquin

&

Denise S. Redmond

professional before attempting any techniques outlined in this book.

By reading this document, the reader agrees that under no circumstances is the author responsible for any losses, direct or indirect, which are incurred as a result of the use of the information contained within this document, including, but not limited to, — errors, omissions, or inaccuracies.

Contents

Ketogenic Vegetarian

101 Delicious Recipes

for a Healthier

Lifestyle and Weight

Loss

Written By

Allyson C. Naquin

INTRODUCTION

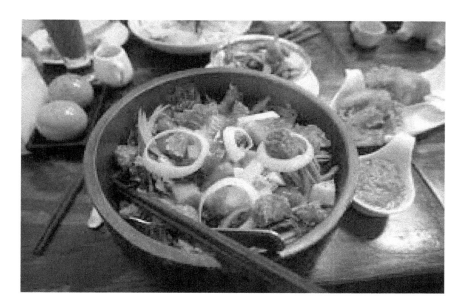

In this book, we will be providing you with healthy and nutritious Vegetarian Keto alternatives and will include recipes that will assist you in reducing the intake of meat. Our main focus is to make the transition to a Keto Vegetarian life much easier for you by creating and presenting a variety of nutritious dishes ranging from easy breakfast recipes to lunch, dinner recipes, snacks and dessert recipes for the whole family.

If you are completely new to vegetarianism, then you may not even know enough about the lifestyle as yet to figure out how you are going to tweak it to be 100%, Keto. This, of course, becomes no easier when you try to do online research as most Keto recipes online are geared towards protein from meat, poultry, or animal products that you may not even eat depending on the category of vegetarian lifestyle you opt to follow.

In this Ketogenic Vegetarian Cookbook, we will be clearing up all those blurry lines. As before you can determine what recipes will be good for you will need to understand what type of vegetarian you will be. There are two main categories in the vegetarian lifestyle that will go more in depth in later on. These are:

- The Vegetarian: A person who does not eat the actual animal but is comfortable eating the by-products that animal may produce. So, for example, people in this category do not eat beef (meat from the cow). However, they may consume dairy products such as milk or cheese that are made from the cow's milk.
- The Vegan: A person who does not eat any animal meat or by-product whatsoever.

There are many different reasons that may lead a person to vegetarianism, and your back story generally influences the type of lifestyle you choose to lead. There are in fact more categories of the lifestyle such as pescatarian, and octo-lacto vegetarian to name a few but for the purposes of this book we will only be focussing on the main two categories.

After we are able to figure out which one of these popular vegetarian categories you will be following, we will then need to move on to helping you understand the keto diet, and how it works. Regardless of the category you select the bases of the Ketogenic diet will still remain the same you will work on getting your body in a state of ketosis while maintaining a healthy, nutrient dense diet. Ketosis occurs when the body produces ketones in your liver that it uses for energy seeing that there is limited starch.

To give you a brief overview, some of the things you are generally privy to enjoying this meal plan are:
- Eggs

- Leafy Greens
- Vegetables that grow above ground
- High Fat Dairy (like Greek yogurt)
- Nuts and seeds
- Avocado and berries
- Natural low-carb sweeteners
- Healthy fats – (like coconut oil, avocado oil, etc.)

You would try to avoid:

- Grains
- Fish or pork that are factory farmed
- Artificial sweeteners
- Refined oils (like canola, and margarine)
- Products labelled low carb, low- fat, or diet
- Milk
- Alcoholic & sweet drinks
- Tropical, high carb fruits (like pineapples, mango, grapes, etc.)
- Juices (even 100% fruit juices)
- Soy products & wheat gluten

Before you dive in any further in food choices, and recipe selection, let's dive in to take a closer look at both the vegetarian, and ketogenic lifestyle so that you can make an informed decision as to what recipes will be best suited for you. While trying to make your decision consider all factors that may affect you in the long run. Here are a few common tips you can help you verify you have made the right decision:

1. Ask yourself do you believe in ethically – A popular determining factor in people opting to go full vegan is their passion for Animal Rights and Cruelty. If you are someone who is really passionate about this, then you probably would not be comfortable on a general vegetarian diet consuming the by-products of animals.

2. Consider any medical conditions you may have – It is always recommended that you consult your physician before opting to select any major lifestyle or dietary change. So, ensure you do all your due dalliance before getting started.

Now that we have covered the bases let's dive right in.

CHAPTER 1:

Vegetarianism

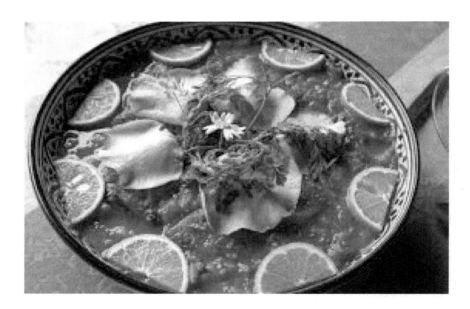

1. What is a Vegetarian?

A vegetarian is a person that has made a conscious decision to avoid animal products in diet or generally speaking, a person who does not eat meat. The main problem in a vegetarian's diet is the lack of protein, of which a gram per kilogram of body mass is needed daily. Also, owing to the fact that humans are omnivores, we lack the appropriate herbivore stomach system that's needed to fully process plants and extract all the nutrients that are within them, so, just eating large quantities of plants will not suffice. Fortunately, there are several types of vegetarian diet, and some of them incorporate eggs, fish or dairy in the diet to make up for the absence of protein. Also, protein powder supplements which were made explicitly for vegetarians can be used.

2. What do you eat as a vegetarian?

Vegetarian foods are so readily available and in huge supply that your meals can never be monotonous are boring. Let's take beans, for example, they are always in such great supply, and there is a wide variety you can eat them everyday of your life without repeating the same meal. Sometimes, your taste buds might be yearning for meat; there is always tofu and other soy products that can be prepared in a way that they look and taste like meat. Your caloric needs can be easily satisfied through vegetarian diet because, many plants store their energy as carbs. However, there is one drawback when proceeding to a keto vegetarian diet.

3. What Is a Vegan?

A vegan is a vegetarian whose diet excludes eggs, meat, dairy products and all other animal by-products. In brief, a vegan is a very moody vegetarian. Being a vegan really means taking the vegetarian diet to another level and discovering new ways to keep away from products that involved suffrage to animals. Your diet should no longer be about just avoiding some types of food but being a relatively conscious consumer that objects to the moral and exploitative nature of the society. For instance, a vegan will strongly object to the consumption of gummy bears, because they are made from gelatin, which prepared by the cooking of pig skin, cow skin, bone, and cartilage. Also, some manufacturers might add gelatin for added thickness to their yogurts and candy, and a vegan will always do their research far in advance.

4. Is it better to be a vegetarian or vegan?

Vegetarian or vegan, which is better? Saying something is better is often subjective especially in this case. A vegetarian aim is to to change his diet; most times for health or moral reasons, where as, a vegan adopts the philosophy of protecting and not harming any living creature and assumes the lifestyle that matches.   A vegetarian will effect change to the diet excluding animal products, but there is a possibility he will continue to wear fur or leather whereas, a vegan will totally avoid animal products, and refuse the wearing of fur or leather and will use neither skin nor hair care products tested on animals.   Whichever one you think is better for you is definitely up to you.

5. What are the Health effects?

Studies on the health effects have shown that vegetarian diets note diverse effects on mortality. One such review found a lower overall risk of all contributes to mortality, cancer (excepting breast) and heart disease; it was analysed by a meta-analysis that it has a lower risk for cancer and ischemic heart disease but no effect at all on overall mortality or cerebrovascular disease. Possible limitations may include many varying definitions used of vegetarianism, plus the observation of the increased risk of lung cancer rate in those persons on a vegetarian diet for a period of five years or less. An analysis done on two large studies revealed that vegetarians in the United Kingdom have a similar cause of mortality as those who eat meat. An earlier meta analysis found the same results, and only found decreased mortality in occasional meat eaters, vegetarians, and pescatarians, in ischemic heart disease, not really from any other cause.

6. Ethics and diet

There is an assortment of ethical motives that leads have been indicated from time to time for selecting vegetarianism, usually dependent on the interests of noninvasive creatures. Some individuals, although not drinkers, refuse to consume the flesh of certain animals due to cultural taboo, like cats, horses, dogs or rabbits. Other people encourage other motives for eating beef such as cultural, scientific, religious and nutritional explanations. Some meat lovers don't consume meat from animals reared in a specific manner, like the ones from factory outlets, they prevent specific meats, like Foie gras or veal. Some men follow vegetarian or vegan diets not from ethical concerns with respect to the increasing or ingestion of creatures generally, but from worries regarding the true therapy and practices that are involved with the raising and slaughter of animals. Some others prevent meat because meat production is believed to put a larger burden on the environment compared to the creation of exactly the exact same quantity of plant protein.

Ethical objections that derive from the account of creatures are divided generally into resistance to the action of murdering generally, and resistance to some agricultural practices encompassing beef production.

7. Religion and diet

An early Indian religion (Jainism) educates vegetarianism as a moral behavior as do some significant sects of Hinduism. Mahayana Buddhism promotes vegetarianism as valuable for growing empathy whereas Buddhism, generally speaking, doesn't prohibit meat consumption. There are different denominations that urge a vegetarian diet these comprise the Seventh-day Adventists, the Rastafari movement, the Ananda Marga movement as well as the Hare Krishnas. Sikhism doesn't compare spirituality with diet and doesn't imply especially a vegetarian or meat diet.

8. Environment and diet

Environmental vegetarianism is the subset of vegetarianism that takes in the farming conditions of the animals into account. It is based primarily on the fact that the mass production of animals and other merchandise solely for consumption is environmentally wrong, especially if done through manufacturing unit farming. In 2006, the United Nations initiative (an international farm animals' enterprise) was identified as one of the most important individuals to environmental degradation. Modern practices which contribute to the raising of animals for food contribute on an "extensive scale" to air and water pollution, land degradation, climate alternate, and loss of biodiversity. The initiative came to an end that "the cattle sector came out as one of the top, or three maximum sizeable members to the maximum extreme environmental problems, at every scale from neighborhood to international."

Additionally, animal agriculture is a massive supply of greenhouse gases. According to a file carried out in 2006, it is liable for 18% of the world's greenhouse fuel emissions as estimated in an one hundred-year CO_2 equivalent. Meat that is produced in a laboratory (known as in vitro meat) can be more environmentally supported than frequently produced meat. Based on the reviews from the Food Climate Research Network at Surrey University it was proven that vegetarian reactions range severely. It's believed that a small variety of animal grazing can be useful for the environment, however, over the years farmers have become to overpack the farms with a large number of animals with limited resources. This often results in a less than ideal situation for both the animals and the environment.

Ghent, Belgium, became pronounced to be "the primary city inside the global in May of 2009 to move vegetarian at the least once every week" for environmental reasons, whilst nearby authorities decided to start a "weekly meatless day." In popularity of the United Nations' record, civil servants might consume vegetarian dishes at some point in every week. Posters were placed up via neighborhood government in popularity to encourage the populace to participate on vegetarian days, and "veggie street maps" have been revealed to highlight vegetarian restaurants. Schools in Ghent are due to have a weekly veggiedag ("vegetarian day") too in September 2009.

CHAPTER 2: The Ketogenic Diet

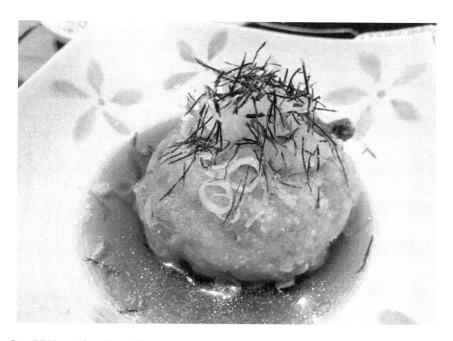

9. What is the Ketogenic diet?

Simply put, the ketogenic diet places a limit on the number of carbohydrates you consume and encourages eating more healthy proteins, and fats. This is to allow your body to enter a state of ketosis forcing your body to use your stored fat for energy instead of your carbs. Of course, it is virtually impossible to completely cut carbohydrates out of your diet, and that is in no way what this diet preaches.

Instead, you are required to limit your total daily carbohydrate intake to 20 grams or less. What this does is force you to make smart decisions regarding what you put in your mouth as you would want to blow this whole allowance on a single candy bar. You will have to bear in mind that certain fruits can also be high in carbohydrates, and you will have to avoid these for the most part as well.

10. Is the Ketogenic diet safe?

Yes, in the large picture of this the Keto diet is a safe lifestyle to follow, with many benefits. However as with another thing in life it also has its share of cons. One of the main disadvantages of the Keto diet is that your diet may be lacking fiber as it is mainly gotten from foods high in carbs. This could potentially lead to constipation issues seeing that the main purpose of fiber in the diet is to help with digestion and waste excretion. To counteract this, you can try adding a bit of crude wheat bran to your diet as its rich in fiber, and relatively low in carbohydrates. Outside of that, there are a few less serious possible side effects including an odor form your sweat, body, and breath.

11. What Do I Eat on a Keto?

When you decide to go on a keto diet, it is vital that you do your required research, and create a plan of action. The first order of business after deciding to switch to a ketogenic diet is trying to get yourself into a state of ketosis. This comes down to how restrictive you can be with the number of carbohydrates each day. The recommended dosage is 20g or less per day. To achieve this, you will have to follow a specific pattern of eating so get rid of the refined carbs such and try to get only healthy carbs from healthy fats and vegetables. Let's look a bit closer on what you should and shouldn't eat as a Ketogenic Vegetarian.

12. Here are some products you can eat freely:

- Animal based proteins – of course as a vegetarian, you won't be eating meat, poultry or fish. So, you will have to get your healthy fatty acids from animal by-products, and other sources. As a vegan, you would not include this category in your diet so

your Omega 3s would mainly be from other food groups, and supplement pills.
- Gelatin
- Pastured eggs
- Butter
- Ghee

- Healthy fats – this category refers to fats you can use to cook your delicious meals with.
  - Goose fat
  - Lard
  - Macadamia oil
  - Tallow
  - Avocado oil
  - Chicken fat
  - Clarified butter or ghee
  - Butter
  - Coconut oil
  - Duck fat
  - Olive oil

- Non-starchy vegetables – not all vegetables are fair game when it comes to a ketogenic diet, as some of them are high in carbs. Here are a few that you can eat as much as you would like.
  - Swiss chard
  - Spinach
  - Radicchio
  - Lettuce
  - Chard
  - Bamboo shoots
  - Radishes
  - Bok choy
  - Chives
  - Endive
  - Spaghetti squash
  - Dark leaf kale
  - Cucumber
  - Kohlrabi
  - Celery stalk
  - Asparagus

- o Zucchini

- Fruits – most fruits, unfortunately, are not a part of the 'eat as much as you want' list, as most fruits have high sugar content. One fruit you can enjoy a lot is:
  - o Avocado

- Beverages and Condiments – when it comes to beverages you want to stay away from anything with artificial sweeteners, additives, soy lecithin, or hormones. Instead, enjoy:
  - o Water
  - o Coffee (sweetened with natural milk or black)
  - o Bone broth
  - o Mustard
  - o Tea (herbal or black)
  - o Mayonnaise
  - o Pesto
  - o Pickles
  - o Kimchi
  - o Kombucha
  - o Sauerkraut
  - o Lime juice and zest
  - o Whey protein

13. Here are foods you can eat occasionally:

- Vegetables, Fruits, and Mushrooms – the vegetables listed below can be eaten only occasionally:
  - o White and green cabbage
  - o Red cabbage
  - o Cauliflower
  - o Broccoli
  - o Brussels sprouts
  - o Fennel
  - o Turnips
  - o Rutabaga
  - o Eggplant
  - o Tomatoes

- Peppers
- Parsley root
- Spring onion
- Leek
- Onion
- Garlic
- Mushrooms
- Pumpkin
- Nori
- Kombu
- Okra
- Bean sprouts
- Sugar snap peas
- Wax beans
- Artichokes
- Water chestnuts
- Rhubarb

- Fruits – as mentioned before most fruits have a high sugar content as such, only certain fruits are allowed to be enjoyed **occasionally** on the keto diet.
  - Blackberries
  - Strawberries
  - Olives
  - Blueberries
  - Raspberries
  - Mulberries
  - Cranberries
  - Coconut

- Dairy (Full – fat) – dairy has always been a grey area when dieting, however, on the Keto diet full fat dairy foods are allowed. Though you have this allowance, you will need to ensure they are all high fat, avoid any products labelled "low – fat" as despite the label they tend to be filled with sugars, starch, and artificial additives. These include:
  - Plain yogurt
  - Cottage cheese
  - Heavy cream
  - Sour cream

- o Cheese

- Seeds, and nuts – you can enjoy seeds, and nuts every now, and again. Below is a list of nuts that can be eaten occasionally to ensure you do not confuse them with legumes.
  - o Hemp seeds
  - o Macadamia nuts
  - o Pecans
  - o Pine nuts
  - o Almonds
  - o Walnuts
  - o Pumpkin seeds
  - o Hazelnuts
  - o Flaxseed
  - o Sesame seeds
  - o Sunflower seeds
  - o Brazil nuts

- Fermented soy products – fermented foods are allowed occasionally if not genetically modified nor processed.
  - o Natto
  - o Tempeh
  - o Black soybeans
  - o Tamari
  - o Coconut aminos
  - o Edamame

- Healthy sweeteners – healthy sweeteners can be used occasionally in place of refined sugars. However, you will have to ensure they are all-natural products.
  - o Stevia
  - o Swerve
  - o Erythritol

- Thickeners – the following thickeners can be used to thicken soups, and sauces occasionally.
  - o Arrowroot powder
  - o Xanthan gum

- Condiments – when it comes to condiments you will have to make a special effort to find sugar-free options that can be had occasionally.
  - Tomato puree
  - Passata
  - Ketchup

- Chocolate, and sweets – in terms of sweets you can enjoy these sugar fee options **that do not have a large number of carbs** occasionally and avoid soy lecithin in the ingredient list. For chocolate, the darker you can get it means the more natural it is. You will need to read the ingredient list.
  - Cocoa
  - Carob powder
  - Chocolate (extra dark)
  - Cocoa powder

- Extras – the following list is a combination of all the lists featured so far. These are all items that you can choose to add in **very small amounts** ONLY if your daily carbohydrate balance allows it. Otherwise, it may be best to avoid them completely.
  - Celery root
  - Carrot
  - Beetroot
  - Parsnip
  - Sweet potato
  - Watermelon
  - Cantaloupe
  - Galia
  - Honeydew melons
  - Pistachio
  - Cashew nuts
  - Chestnuts
  - Apricot
  - Dragon fruit
  - Peach
  - Nectarine
  - Apple
  - Grapefruit

- ○ Kiwifruit
- ○ Kiwi berries
- ○ Orange
- ○ Plums
- ○ Cherries
- ○ Pears
- ○ Figs

This goes without saying, however, the only way you will be able to tell what your carbohydrates levels are to decide whether or not you can allow one of these items is to maintain a realistic food journal. This journal should include information about everything you are eating and should be as accurate as possible. As time goes by you will be able to estimate, and determine what to have off the top of your head, however, when you are just transitioning to a keto diet keeping a journal is highly recommended.

Now that we have explored detailed explanations of both vegetarianism and the ketogenic lifestyle let's dive in to some actual recipes that you will be able to use to help you on your way. Enjoy!

CHAPTER 3: Breakfast Recipes

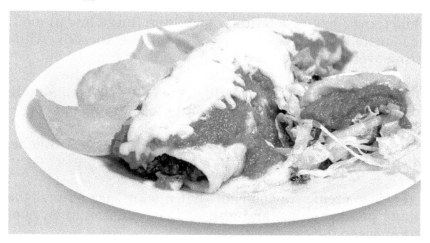

Thank you for allowing us to expose you to the large variety of Keto Vegetarian recipes that you can enjoy, please feel free to leave us a positive review if you like what you are about to read through.

1. Pesto Scrambled Eggs

Yield: 1 Servings
Total Time: 10 Minutes
Prep Time: 5 Minutes
Cook Time: 5 Minutes

Ingredients
- Eggs (3 large, free-range)
- Butter (1 tbsp.)
- Pesto (1 tbsp.)
- Crème fraîche (2 tbsp.)
- Salt (to taste)

- Black pepper (to taste)

Directions

Add your eggs to a mixing bowl then season with salt and pepper. Whisk until fully beaten (should be frothy). Next, set a skillet, over low heat, with your butter, and allow to melt. Once melted, add eggs, stir, and continue to cook while stirring over low heat.

Note: Stirring the eggs constantly helps the eggs to maintain a creamy texture, and stops them from fully drying out.

Stir in your pesto then remove from heat. Add crème fraiche, and stir well to fully incorporate.

Note: The crème fraiche cools down your eggs so that the cooking process stops, and also adds an additional layer of creaminess to the eggs.

Serve with avocados, or keto approved buns!

Nutritional Information per Serving:

Calories: 468; Total Fat: 42 g; Carbs: 3.3 g; Dietary Fiber: 0.7 g; Sugars: 0 g; Protein: 20.4 g; Cholesterol: 0 mg; Sodium: 0 mg

2. Baby Kale, Mozzarella, and Egg Bake

Yield: 6 Servings
Total Time: 51 Minutes
Prep Time: 15 Minutes
Cook Time: 36 Minutes

Ingredients
- Kale (5 oz., dark, chopped)
- Olive oil (2 tsp.)
- Mozzarella cheese (1½ cup, low-fat, grated)
- Green onion (1/3 cup, thinly sliced)
- Eggs (8)
- Spike seasoning (1 tsp.)
- Salt and pepper to taste

Directions
Set your oven to 375 degrees F, and prepare a casserole dish by lightly greasing with olive oil cooking spray, and set aside. While that heats up, set a skillet with olive oil over medium heat and allow to get hot. Add kale, and cook, while stirring, until wilted (about 3 minutes). Once wilted add to your prepared casserole dish, and spread to cover the bottom of the dish.

Top your kale with onions, and cheese. Crack eggs into a medium bowl, and season to taste with pepper, Spike seasoning, and salt. Whisk to fully combine, then pour in your casserole dish over the kale, onions, and cheese. Stir gently to evenly combine then set to bake in your preheated oven.

Allow to bake until the egg as become completely set, and lightly golden brown (about 35 minutes). Remove from oven, cool slightly, slice, and serve.

Nutritional Information per Serving:
Calories: 124; Total Fat: 8 g; Carbs: 4 g; Dietary Fiber: 1 g;
Sugars: 1 g; Protein: 10.2 g; Cholesterol: 222 mg; Sodium: 136
mg

3. **Pesto Egg Muffins**

Yield: 10 Servings
Total Time: 30 Minutes
Prep Time: 5 Minutes
Cook Time: 25 Minutes

Ingredients

- Spinach (⅔ cup, frozen, thawed, drained)
- Pesto (3 tbsp.)
- Kalamata olives (½ cup, pitted)
- Sun-dried tomatoes (¼ cup, chopped)
- Goat cheese (125g., soft)
- Eggs (6 large, free-range)
- Salt (to taste)
- Pepper (to taste)

Directions

Set your oven to preheat to 350 degrees F, and prepare a muffin tin by fitting it with paper muffin cups. Drain as much liquid from your thawed spinach as possible and set aside. Slice olives, and discard seeds then aside. Roughly chop your sun-dried tomatoes. Add your eggs, and pesto into a medium bowl then season to taste with pepper and salt. Whisk until fully combined.

Evenly split your olives, chopped tomato, crumbled goat cheese, and spinach in your muffin cups. Top each cup evenly with your pesto egg mixture and set in preheated oven to bake. Allow to bake until eggs are fully set, and the tops become lightly browned (about 25 minutes). Remove from heat, allow to cool slightly, and serve.

Nutritional Information per Serving:

Calories: 125; Total Fat: 10.2 g; Carbs: 2 g; Dietary Fiber: 1 g; Sugars: 1 g; Protein: 7 g; Cholesterol: 123 mg; Sodium: 193 mg

4. <u>**Cheesy Egg Muffins**</u>

Yield: 6 Servings
Total Time: 30 Minutes
Prep Time: 10 Minutes
Cook Time: 20 Minutes

Ingredients
- Eggs (4 large)
- Greek yogurt (2 tbsp., full fat)
- Salt (to taste)
- Coconut flour (3 tbsp.)
- Baking powder (¼ tsp.)
- Cheddar cheese (½ cup, shredded)
- Black pepper (to taste)

Directions
Set your oven to preheat to 375 degrees F. Add yogurt, and eggs to a medium bowl, season with salt, and pepper, then whisk to combine. Add your baking powder, and coconut flour, then mix to form a smooth batter. Finally, add your cheese, and fold to combine. Pour your mixture evenly into 6 silicone muffin cups and set to bake in your preheated oven.

Note: If you do not have silicone muffin cups, line your metal muffin tin with paper cups, and lightly grease your paper muffin cups with olive oil.

Allow to bake until your eggs are fully set, and lightly golden on top (about 20 minutes, turning the tray at the halfway point). Allow muffins to cool on a cooling rack then serve. Enjoy!

Nutritional Information per Serving:
Calories: 101; Total Fat: 7 g; Carbs: 3 g; Dietary Fiber: 1.5; Sugars: 0.3 g; Protein: 7 g; Cholesterol: 134 mg; Sodium: 132 mg

5. Skillet-Baked Eggs with Spinach, Yogurt, and Chili Oil

Yield: 4 Servings
Total Time: 40 Minutes
Prep Time: 10 Minutes
Cook Time: 30 Minutes

Ingredients
- Greek yogurt (2/3 cup, plain)
- Garlic (1 clove, halved)
- Salt (to taste)
- Butter (2 tbsp., unsalted)
- Olive oil (2 tbsp.)
- Leek (3 tbsp., chopped)
- Green onions (2 tbsp., chopped)
- Spinach (10 cups, fresh leaves)
- Lemon juice (1 tsp.)
- Eggs (4 large)
- Red pepper flakes (1/4 tsp., crushed)
- Paprika (1/4 tsp.)
- Oregano (1 tsp., chopped)

Directions
Set your oven to preheat to 300 degrees F. In a medium bowl, combine garlic, and yogurt, season with salt, and pepper then whisk to combine. Set aside. Set a skillet with half of your butter, and oil over medium heat to get hot. Add scallion, and leek; switch heat to low. Allow to cook for 10 minutes (or until soft). Add lemon juice, and spinach then season to taste with salt. Turn up your heat to medium, and cook, while stirring, until wilted (about 5 minutes). Remove from heat.

Carefully drain any excess liquid from your spinach, and transfer it to another large skillet. Spread the spinach so that

4 deep wells are created. Add an egg to each well, and carefully set to bake in the preheated oven. Allow to bake for about 15 minutes (or until egg white are fully cooked).

Set a sauce pan with your remaining butter over medium heat, and allow to melt. Once melted, stir in paprika, pepper flakes, and salt. Allow to cook for about a minute (or until butter is browned, and foamy). Stir in oregano and cook for another 30 seconds. Remove from heat.

Discard garlic from yogurt mixture. Serve your baked egg with spinach, topped with a spoon of garlic yogurt, and a drizzle of spicy butter. Enjoy!

Nutritional Information per Serving:
Calories:219; Total Fat: 18 g; Carbs: 6 g; Dietary Fiber: 2 g; Sugars: 2 g; Protein: 11 g; Cholesterol: 201 mg; Sodium: 221 mg

6. <u>Eggs Baked in Avocado Recipe</u>

Yield: 4 Servings
Total Time: 25 Minutes
Prep Time: 15 Minutes
Cook Time: 10 Minutes

Ingredients
- Avocados (4)
- Eggs (8)
- Limes (2)
- Salt, and pepper (to taste)
- Cilantro (1 tbsp., chopped)
- Scallions (1 tbsp., chopped)
- Chilies (1, sliced)

Directions
Reposition your oven rack so that it is in the middle of your oven, then set your oven to preheat to 450 degrees F. Prepare avocado by slicing avocados in half lengthwise, and discarding the seeds. Make each avocado hallow enough to hold an egg, by scooping out some of the flesh from the center.

Drizzle each avocado half with lime juice, and season lightly with salt. Place your avocados skin side down on a lined baking sheet then crack an egg into each avocado half. Set to bake in your preheated oven for about 12 minutes (until egg whites are fully set). When done, remove from heat, and top evenly with your remaining ingredients. Enjoy!

Nutritional Information per Serving:
Calories: 546; Total Fat: 48 g; Carbs: 22 g; Dietary Fiber: 14 g; Sugars: 2.3 g; Protein: 15.1 g; Cholesterol: 327 mg; Sodium: 136 mg

7. <u>**Savory Crepes**</u>

Yield: 2 Servings
Total Time: 15 Minutes
Prep Time: 5 Minutes
Cook Time: 10 Minute

Ingredients
<u>Crepes:</u>
- Eggs (4)
- Almond milk (¼ cup, unsweetened)
- Coconut flour (1 tbsp.)
- Salt (¼ tsp)
- Parsley (¼ cup, finely chopped)
- Coconut oil for frying

<u>Filling ideas:</u>
- Avocado (1, peeled, diced)

Directions
Combine all your crepe ingredients into a medium bowl, then whisk until a smooth batter is formed. Allow the mixture to stand like this for about 10 minutes to thicken a little.

Note: If you plan to create ahead of time to create these crepes for breakfast, consider creating the batter from the night before, cover, and store in the refrigerator overnight. That way your batter will be ready for you when you wake up in the morning.

Set a large greased skillet over medium heat to get hot. Stir the batter, and add a few tablespoons of the batter to the center of your hot skillet. Swirl the skillet so that the batter spreads and creates a thin layer over the bottom of the skillet. Allow to cook for about 2 minutes, or until golden brown. Transfer from heat to a serving plate, top diced avocado, roll and serve.

Nutritional Information per Serving:
Calories: 146; Total Fat: 10 g; Carbs: 3.4 g; Dietary Fiber: 1.6 g; Sugars: 0.7 g; Protein: 12 g; Cholesterol: 327 mg; Sodium: 190 mg

8. **Egg Stuffed Avocado**

Yield: 2 Servings
Total Time: 15 Min.
Prep Time: 5 Min.
Cook Time: 10 Min.

Ingredients

- Avocado (1 extra-large, seeded)
- Eggs (4 large, free-range)
- Mayonnaise (¼ cup)
- Sour cream (2 tbsp.)
- Dijon mustard (1 tsp.)
- Spring onions (2 medium)
- Salt (to taste)
- Black pepper (to taste)

Directions

Set a small saucepan with enough water to fill ¾ of the pan. Season water with salt, and allow to come to a boil.
Note: Cooking eggs in salted water prevents the eggs from cracking under the pressure of the water.
Gently add your eggs to your boiling water with a spoon. Allow eggs to cook for about 10 minutes to achieve a hard-boiled egg. Switch off heat and carefully transfer your eggs to a bowl of ice water with a slotted spoon. Allow to cool down. Once cool, peel the shell from the eggs.
Dice your eggs, and add to a medium bowl. Scoop out about a tablespoon of avocado flesh from the center of each half, dice, and add to eggs. Add spring onions, sour cream, Dijon mustard, and mayo. Season to taste with pepper, and salt. Stir to combine, and spoon the mixture evenly back into your avocado halves. Serve, and enjoy!

Nutritional Information per Serving:

Calories: 616; Total Fat: 57 g; Carbs: 15 g; Dietary Fiber: 10 g; Sugars: 3.5 g; Protein: 16.5 g; Cholesterol: 385 mg; Sodium: 683 mg

9. <u>Egg and Nori Rolls</u>

Yield: 4 Servings
Total Time: 25 Minutes
Prep Time:10 Minutes
Cook Time: 15 Minutes

Ingredients

- Soy sauce (3 tablespoons)
- Water (1/2 cup)
- Salt (1/4 tsp.)
- Sushi nori (4 sheets)
- Celery sticks (2, sliced into matchsticks)
- Wasabi paste (1/2 teaspoon)
- Eggs (8, room temp)
- Olive oil (1 tablespoon)
- Carrot (1, sliced into matchsticks)
- Snow peas sprouts (1/2 cup, stems removed)

Directions

Using a small bowl mix together ¼ cup water, soy sauce, and wasabi. Put aside till needed. Put eggs in a bowl along with leftover water and salt. Whisk to combine.

Heat a teaspoon of oil in frying pan and pour in ¼ of an egg; tilt pan to spread egg all over the bottom of the pan.

Cook for 2 minutes then remove from pan. Repeat with remaining egg.

Place each cooked egg flat and place nori on top. Put vegetables in the middle and roll. Cut in half and serve with wasabi.

Nutritional Information per Serving:

Calories: 80; Total Fat: 6 g; Carbs: 3 g; Dietary Fiber: 1 g; Sugars: 1.3 g; Protein: 4 g; Cholesterol: 155 mg; Sodium: 947 mg

10. Grilled Avocado with Melted Cheese & Hot Sauce

Yield: 1 Servings
Total Time: 9 Minutes
Prep Time: 5 Minutes
Cook Time: 4 Minutes

Ingredients
- Avocado (1)
- Chipotle sauce (1 tbsp.)
- Lime juice (1 tbsp.)
- Parmesan cheese (¼ cup)
- Salt (to taste)
- Pepper (to taste)

Directions
Prepare your avocado by slicing it in half lengthwise, and discarding the seed. Gently prick the skin of your avocado with a fork randomly, and set aside.

Note: Pricking the skin of the avocado will allow for your sauce to properly penetrate the avocado's flesh later in the recipe.

Set your avocado halves, skin side down, on a small baking sheet, line with aluminum foil. Top evenly with your sauce, then drizzle with lime juice. Season to taste with pepper, and salt.

Sprinkle a half parmesan cheese in each cavity, and set your broiler on high for 2 minutes. Add your remaining parmesan cheese, and return to the broiler until cheese completely melts, and avocado slightly browns (about another 2 minutes). Serve hot, with a side of extra chipotle sauce.

Nutritional Information per Serving:
Calories: 459; Total Fat: 41 g; Carbs: 24 g; Dietary Fiber: 14 g;
Sugars: 5 g; Protein: 6.3 g; Cholesterol: 5 mg; Sodium: 138 mg

11. <u>**Eggs Florentine**</u>

Yield: 1 Servings
Total Time: 8 Minutes
Prep Time: 3 Minutes
Cook Time: 5 Minutes

Ingredients:
- 2 large eggs (2 large)
- extra virgin olive oil (1 tbsp., unfiltered)
- Egg Fast Alfredo Sauce (5 tbsp.)
- Organic Parmigiano Reggiano Wedge (1 tbsp., divided)
- organic baby spinach (3 grams)
- red pepper flakes (1 pinch)

Directions:
Set oven rack in the top groove nearest to the broiler. Set broiler to preheat.

Place olive oil in a non-stick skillet and put to heat over medium high heat. Gently, fry eggs over medium flame, until egg whites are opaque but the yolk still runny. This takes roughly 4 mins. Do not turn over eggs. Prepare casserole in the meantime.

Dribble some olive oil in each casserole container or spray with cooking spray (olive oil).

In the bottom of the casserole, spread half of the Alfredo sauce. Slide gently, the half-done egg atop sauce. Spread leftover Alfredo sauce and half of the parmesan cheese over eggs.

Set casserole under the broiler and broil for 2-3 mins or until the eggs have formed and the top has bubbly golden spots. Remove from broiler and top with thinly sliced (julienne) baby spinach leaves, unused Parmesan cheese and a dash of red pepper flakes. Serve instantly.

Nutritional Information per Serving:
Calories: 529; Total Fat: 49 g; Carbs: 3 g; Dietary Fiber: 1 g;
Sugars: 4 g; Protein: 20 g; Cholesterol: 490 mg; Sodium: 479
mg

CHAPTER 4: Lunch Recipes

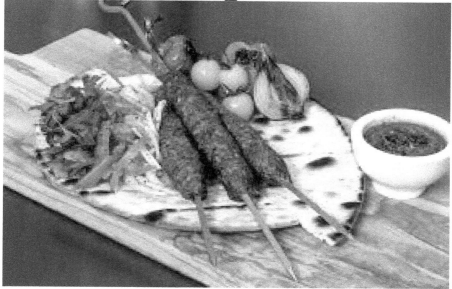

Thank you for allowing us to expose you to the large variety of Keto Vegetarian recipes that you can enjoy, please feel free to leave us a positive review if you like what you are about to read through.

12. Garlic Parmesan Fried Eggplant

Yield: 6 Servings
Total Time: 21 Minutes
Prep Time: 15 Minutes
Cook Time: 6 Minutes

Ingredients
- Eggplant (1 medium)

- Salt (1/2 tsp.)
- Egg (1 large)
- Almond flour (1 cup)
- Parmesan cheese (1 cup, grated)
- Garlic powder (2 tsp.)
- Salt (to taste)
- Pepper (to taste)
- Coconut oil (1/4 cup)

Directions

Prepare eggplant by slicing into thick slices. Lay your slices on a flat surface then blot with a hand towel to remove excess water. Season with salt, and allow to marinate for about 30 minutes. Blot, once more to remove any water that may have pooled up.

Blot eggplant dry with a paper towel. Add eggs to a medium bowl, and whisk until well beaten. Add garlic powder, parmesan cheese, and almond flour to a large bowl. Season with pepper, and salt, and stir to combine.

Set a skillet with coconut oil to get hot, over medium heat. Add your eggplant slices to your egg bowl. Use a pair of tongs to lift out, gently shake off any excess egg drippings, then dredge into flour mixture. Lift out and add to the hot skillet to fry until browned on all sides and crispy. Repeat the process until all your eggplant has been cooked.

Nutritional Information per Serving:

Calories: 271; Total Fat: 22 g; Carbs: 10 g; Dietary Fiber: 3.4 g; Sugars: 0.77 g; Protein: 12 g; Cholesterol: 67 mg; Sodium: 696 mg

13. Low-Carb Thin Crust White Pizza

Yield: 2-4 Servings
Total time: 45 Minutes
Prep time: 10 Minutes
Cook time: 2 Hours

Ingredients
Crust:
- almond flour (1/2 cup)
- egg white protein powder (¼ cup)
- parmesan cheese (1/2 cup, grated)
- organic egg (1 large)
- sea salt (1/4 tsp. or more to taste)

Topping:
- cream cheese (2 tbsp.)
- cream (1 tbsp., heavy whipping)
- onion powder (1 tsp.)
- feta cheese (1/2 cup, crumbled)
- hard cheese (1/2 cup, grated)
- red onion (1 small, peeled and sliced))
- Kalamata olives (1/4 cup, seedless, chopped)
- olive oil (1 tbsp. extra virgin)

Directions
Heat oven to 200 degrees C. In a bowl, place all the dry ingredients needed for the crust and mix well. Add the egg and knead with your hands. Line a medium skillet with parchment paper.

Use a rolling pin or your fingers to spread evenly into a thin batter. Wet your fingers to prevent the batter from sticking to them. Bake into the oven for a period of 10 to 15 mins. until slightly golden. Prepare white sauce in the meanwhile by combining cream and onion powder thoroughly.

Remove crust from the oven when it is done and cover top with white sauce. Add grated cheese, crumbled feta, olives, and onions, bake for a further 10 mins. Take out of the oven when completed and use a sharp knife or pizza cutter to cut the pizza into quarters. Garnish with fresh rocket leaves drizzled with olive oil. Put on a serving plate. Enjoy!

Nutritional Information per Serving:
Calories: 352; Total Fat: 29 g; Carbs: 7 g; Dietary Fiber: 2.1 g; Sugars: 7.3 g; Protein: 20g; Cholesterol: 313 mg; Sodium: 563 mg

14.<u>Creamy Kale Salad</u>

Yield: 3 Servings
Total Time: 10 Minutes
Prep Time: 10 Minutes
Cook Time: 0 Minutes

Ingredients
- 1 bunch kale
- 1 bunch spinach
- 1 cup sour cream
- 1 cup roasted macadamia
- ½ cup parmesan cheese, grated
- 1 garlic clove, minced
- ¼ teaspoon salt
- 2 tablespoons lime juice
- ½ teaspoon black pepper
- 2 tablespoons sesame seeds oil
- 1 tbsp. lemon juice

<u>Toppings</u>

Pecans (1/4 cup, chopped)
Avocado (1 1/2, diced)
Goat Cheese (3 oz.)

Directions
Chop kale and wash kale then remove the ribs. Transfer kale to a large bowl. Add sour cream, macadamia, lime juice, sesame seeds oil, pepper, salt, garlic and grated cheese. Mix thoroughly. Top with your goat cheese, avocado, and pecans. Serve and enjoy.

Nutritional Information per Serving:
Calories: 78; Total Fat: 6.4 g; Carbs: 3.2 g; Dietary Fiber: 2.2 g; Sugars: 3.2 g; Protein: 1.1 g; Cholesterol: 9.9 mg; Sodium: 172 mg

15. **Vegetarian Keto Burgers**

Yield: 2 Servings
Total time: 20 Minutes
Prep time: 5 Minutes
Cook time:15 minutes

Ingredients
- flat mushrooms (2 large, chopped)
- coconut oil (3 tsp.)
- dried basil (1 tsp.)
- dried oregano or (½ tsp.)
- garlic (1 clove, crushed)
- black pepper (freshly ground)
- keto buns (2)
- 2 eggs
- cheddar cheese (2 slices)
- mayo (2 tbsp.)
- lettuce for garnishing

Directions
Season mushroom with crushed garlic, basil, oregano, 1 tsp. oil, salt, and pepper. Rub in seasoning and leave to marinate for roughly 1 hour. Mushrooms should be kept at room temperature. Marinating is highly recommended, but if you are pressed for time, you can skip this process.

On a hot griddle or regular pan place mushrooms with the top-side up and cook for 5 mins. over medium high heat. Remove from heat. Flip mushrooms back on the top -side. Just before you are ready to serve, place slices of cheese on top of mushrooms and broil until cheese melts. In the meantime, heat remaining 2 tsp. of oil. Fry eggs individually until egg white is hard and the yolk runny (this creates a perfect shape for the burgers); remove from the heat.

Split buns into halves. On a hot griddle pan, place the cut side down and cook until crispy.Apply 1 tbsp. mayo on each bun half; add mushrooms; topped with fried eggs and lettuce. Enjoy!

Nutritional Information per Serving:
Calories: 637; Total Fat: 10 g; Carbs: 19 g; Dietary Fiber: 10.1 g; Sugars: 4 g; Protein: 24g; Cholesterol: 10 mg; Sodium: 0 mg

16. **Broccoli Crust Pizza**

Yield: 2 Servings
Total Time: 35 Minutes
Prep Time: 10 Minutes
Cook Time: 25 Minutes

Ingredients
- mushrooms (3 large, sliced)
- onion (2 small, minced)
- carrots (2 cubed)
- turnip (1 small, cubed)
- chayote (1, cubed)
- celery (2 stalks, cubed)
- tin corn (1- 14 oz)
- garlic (4 cloves, diced)
- ginger (2 inches, crushed)
- bay leaves (3)
- turmeric (1/4 tsp.)
- black pepper (1 tsp.)
- Pinch of salt

Directions
Heat your oven to 200 degrees C. Pulse onion and broccoli in a food mixer until chopped finely. Add balance of ingredients and pulse until all are chopped and thoroughly combined. Put aside the mixture for 15 mins., this will allow the liquid to be absorbed by the chia seeds and husk.

Use your fingers or a roller to form the pizza on a baking tray covered with parchment paper. Spread pizza in the same thickness right around, so it bakes evenly. Bake for a 10 minute period then flip it gently over and bake for a further 5 mins.

Remove pizza crust from oven and add the desired topping. Here are some suggestions: organic tomato puree, chili powder, a small amount of garlic powder, fresh basil, goat cheese, paprika, sliced tomato and onion rings. Bake pizzas for an additional 5 mins. then remove. Add arugula and a little fresher basil and serve.

Nutritional Information per Serving:
Calories: 248; Total Fat: 1.5 g; Carbs: 60 g; Dietary Fiber: 9 g; Sugars: 16 g; Protein: 8 g; Cholesterol: 0 mg; Sodium: 602 mg

17. <u>Low Carb Falafel with Tahini Sauce</u>

Yield: 8 Servings
Total Time: 27 Minutes
Prep Time: 10 Minutes
Cook Time: 20 Minutes

Ingredients
- raw cauliflower (1 cup, pureed)
- ground slivered almonds (1/2 cup)
- ground cumin (1 tbsp.)
- Tbsp ground coriander (1 ½ tsp.)
- kosher salt (1 tsp.)
- cayenne pepper (½ tsp.)
- garlic, minced (1 clove)
- fresh parsley (2 tbsp, chopped)
- 2 large eggs (2 large)
- 3 Tbsp coconut flour
- Tahini sauce:
- tahini paste (2 tbsp.)
- water (2 tbsp.)
- lemon juice (1 tsp)
- garlic (1 clove, minced)
- kosher salt, more to taste if desired

Directions

First, we will make a cup of cauliflower puree. Using 1 medium head of cauliflower (only florets); chop up using a knife, place in a food blender (processor or magic bullet). Pulse until blended but leaving grainy texture. You can grind the almonds in a similar manner but be careful not to over grind.

In a medium bowl, blend together the grounded cauliflower and almonds. Add all other ingredients and stir until everything is combined. Put to heat a half and half mix of any light oil (grapeseed and olive oil are fine) until it's sizzling. During that process, arrange the mixture into eight 3-inch patties that are roughly the same thickness of a hockey puck.

Fry four first until both sides are browned, then fry the remaining four. Don't flip too soon; you want to see the edges a nice rich brown before you attempt to. Give it about 3-4 mins. on each side. Transfer to a lined plate (can use a paper towel to the line), to absorb excess oil. Serve these with the tahini sauce and garnish as desired.

Tahini sauce: In a small bowl, blend all ingredients together. Thin with a little more water if you prefer a lighter consistency.

Nutritional Information per Serving:
Calories: 281; Total Fat: 24 g; Carbs: 5 g; Dietary Fiber: 4 g; Sugars: 4 g; Protein: 8 g; Cholesterol: 386 mg; Sodium: 1131mg

18. <u>Stuffed Eggplant</u>

Yield: 6 Servings
Total Time: 1 Hour 35 Minutes
Prep Time: 15 Minutes
Cook Time: 1 Hour 20 Minutes

Ingredients

- eggplants (6 slender, preferably Japanese eggplants)
- olive oil (4 tbsp., divided)
- red onions (2 medium, chopped)
- garlic (4 cloves, minced)
- fresh parsley (3 tbsp., chopped)
- bell pepper (1 green, seeded and chopped)
- tomatoes (4, chopped)
- raw coconut palm sugar (1 tsp.)
- ground cumin (1 tsp.)
- tomato paste (1 tbsp.)
- salt (to taste)
- black pepper (to taste)

Directions

Place a rack in the middle of the oven and preheat to 230 degrees C (450 degrees F).
Use aluminum foil or parchment paper to line baking tray then brush it with some olive oil. Remove wide strips from the skin of the eggplants. A vegetable peeler should be used.

Using a vegetable peeler, remove wide strips of the eggplants' skin. Split the eggplants in a lengthwise direction, careful not to slice straight through them. In each eggplant, sprinkle a generous pinch of salt, leave them in a colander to rest for about half an hour.

Place eggplants on the lined baking tray, bake for 20 minutes or until the outer skin begins shriveling. When completed, remove and set aside. Set a skillet over medium heat, add 2 tbsp. of oil and onions then sauté until soft. Add the bell pepper and garlic.

Continue cooking for another 10 mins., until the vegetables are soft. Use salt and pepper to season, mix in the sugar, chopped tomato, cumin, parsley and tomato paste, and parsley. Cook for 5 mins, until the fragrance, permeates the air. Set aside.
Reduce the temperature in the oven to 180 degrees C (350 degrees F). Lay each eggplant in the baking dish so that it opens up like a butterfly. Fill it with the tomato and onion mixture. Drizzle with the remaining portion of olive oil, then add 6 tsp. of water and bake for 40 to 45 minutes.

When cooking is completed, the eggplants should be flat and the liquid in the pan a slight resemblance of honey. Serve at room temperature, and spoon some of the liquid from the pan over the eggplant.

Nutritional Information per Serving:
Calories: 116; Total Fat: 12 g; Carbs: 11 g; Dietary Fiber: 20 g; Sugars: 24 g; Protein: 3 g; Cholesterol: 0 mg; Sodium: 24 mg

19. Buffalo "Potato" Wedges with Blue Cheese Drizzle

Yield: 4 Servings
Total Time: 1 Hour
Prep Time: 15 Minutes
Cook Time: 45 Minutes

Ingredients
- rutabagas (2 medium, cleaned and peeled)
- butter (4 tbsp.)
- salt (1/2 tsp)
- onion powder (1/2 tsp.)
- black pepper (1/8 tsp.)
- buffalo wing sauce (1/2 cup)
- blue cheese dressing (1/4 cup)
- green onions (2, chopped)

Directions
Heat oven to 400 degrees F and use parchment paper to line baking sheet.

Wash and peel the rutabagas Clean and peel rutabagas and cut into a wedge shape.

On low heat, melt butter and stir in onion powder, salt, onion, and black pepper. Use seasoned melted butter to coat wedge shaped rutabaga liberally. Arrange layer singly on a baking sheet. Bake for half of an hour.

Remove for a short while from oven; coat in buffalo wing sauce. Return to oven and bake for a further 15 mins. Place wedges on a serving plate and trickle with blue cheese dressing. Garnish with chopped green onion on top. Serve.

Nutritional Information per Serving:
Calories: 235; Total Fat: 15 g; Carbs: 10 g; Dietary Fiber: 5.4 g; Sugars: 11 g; Protein: 2.5 g; Cholesterol: 23 mg; Sodium: 505 mg

20. <u>Italian-Style Baked Mushrooms</u>

Yield: 3-4 Servings
Prep Time: 15 Minutes
Cook Time: 30 Minutes
Total Time: 45 Minutes

Ingredients
- Portobello mushrooms (1 lb.)
- canned tomatoes (1 large, unsweetened)
- parmesan cheese (2 cups, grated)
- garlic /onion ghee (2 tbsp.)
- basil (2 tbsp., fresh)
- parsley (1 tbsp., fresh)
- oregano (1 tsp. dried)
- salt and pepper to taste

Directions
Heat oven to 400 degrees F / 200 degrees C. Clean mushrooms and slice.
In a non-stick pan, heat the garlic-infused ghee over medium flame. Put in sliced mushrooms, add salt and pepper to taste. Heat the garlic ghee in a non-stick saucepan over medium flame. Add the mushrooms, mix in salt and pepper and sauté for roughly 5 minutes.

Remove saucepan from flame and arrange the mushrooms on small baking containers.
Wash and chop basil, parsley, and oregano. In a medium sized bowl, combine the parsley, basil, oregano and canned tomatoes and add salt to taste. Sprinkle with grated cheese and bake in the oven within 20-25 minutes. When completed, remove with caution from the oven. Allow to cool for a couple minutes on a cooling rack.

Nutritional Information per Serving:

Calories: 232; Total Fat: 16 g; Carbs: 10.3 g; Dietary Fiber: 3 g; Sugars: 2.1 g; Protein: 15 g; Cholesterol: 43 mg; Sodium: 906 mg

21. <u>Tofu Taco Salad</u>

Yield: 4 Servings
Total Time: 40 Minutes
Prep Time: 10 Minutes
Cook Time: 30 Minutes

Ingredients
- Tofu (1 lb., extra firm, drained, sliced into triangles)

Spice Blend:
- Water (1 cup, water)
- Paprika (1 teaspoon)
- Onion Powder (1 tablespoon)
- Chili powder (1 tablespoon)
- Salt (1/2 teaspoon)
- Dried oregano (2 teaspoons)
- Ground cumin (1 tablespoon)

Salad:
- Black olives (1 can cut)
- Spinach (12 oz.)
- Red Onions (1 medium, sliced)
- Red Bell Pepper (1 large, cored, seeded & sliced)

Dressing:
- Tomato sauce (3/4 cup)
- Avocado (1)
- Lime (1/2 juiced)

Directions
Use a large skillet to cook tofu until browned. Combine all seasonings in a bowl and add water; whisk mixture together. Pour mixture onto tofu and cook for about 15 minutes until liquid has reduced. Blend tomato juice, avocado, and lime juice until smooth. Place salad greens in a container and top with black olives, red onions, red pepper, tofu, chickpeas, and dressing. Serve and enjoy!

Nutritional Information per Serving: Calories: 379.5; Total Fat: 14 g; Carbs: 22.75 g; Dietary Fiber: 4.5 g; Sugars: 3 g; Protein: 21.75 g; Cholesterol: 0 mg; Sodium: 449 mg

22. <u>Eggplant Hole in the Head</u>

Yield: 3 Servings
Total Time: 30 Minutes
Prep Time: 10 Minutes
Cook Time: 20 Minutes

Ingredients
- Eggplant (1 whole)
- Extra Virgin Olive Oil (1 tbsp.)
- salted butter (1 tbsp.)
- pastured eggs (4 whole)
- black pepper (1 tsp.)
- salt (1 tsp.)

Directions
Prepare and heat grill to high heat. Wash eggplant, from one end to the other, cut into thick slices (1"). Coat the slices from the eggplant with olive oil and apply a dash of salt.
Place eggplant on grill and cook for four mins. per side.

For each piece of eggplant, cut a hole in the center with a circular cookie cutter. Prepare medium heat and sauté eggplant in a frying pan with the pasture butter. Break an egg into the center of each slice of eggplant. Allow 3-4 mins. for the egg to cook and then flip cautiously.

Cook for a further 3 mins, adding salt and pepper to desired taste. Garnish with sliced green pepper and serve.

Nutritional Information per Serving:
Calories: 247; Total Fat: 16 g; Carbs: 13 g; Dietary Fiber: 6 g; Sugars: 7.3 g; Protein: 14 g; Cholesterol: 828 mg; Sodium: 962 mg

23. Avocado with Broccoli and Zucchini Salad

Yield: 2 Servings
Total Time: 20 Minutes
Prep Time: 10 Minutes
Cook Time: 10 Minutes

Ingredients
- 2 large zucchinis, julienne
- 2 tablespoons tamari sauce
- ¼ teaspoon salt
- 1 cup broccoli, cut into florets
- 1 avocado, sliced
- ½ cup sun dried tomatoes
- ½ cup basil leaves
- 1 teaspoon black pepper
- 1 tablespoon apple cider vinegar

Directions
To create zucchini noodles (zoodles) using a vegetable peeler, shave the zucchini with the peeler lengthwise until you get to the core with the seeds. Turn the zucchini, and repeat the process is creating long strips. Continue repeating the process until you have shaved all the zucchini into strips, and discard the seeds. Now lay your strips on a cutting board, and slice lengthwise to the desired thickness that you would like your zoodle to be.

Tip: Alternately this process could also be done using a spiralizer, mandolin, or julienne peeler.

Combine zucchini, dried tomatoes, broccoli, vinegar, salt, pepper, tamari sauce, and mix well. Place avocado slices and basil on top, serve. Enjoy.

Nutritional Information per Serving:

Calories: 159; Total Fat: 8.4 g; Carbs: 28 g; Dietary Fiber: 19 g; Sugars: 6.2 g; Protein:8 g; Cholesterol: 0 mg; Sodium: 466 mg

24. Onion & Zucchini Salad Bowl

Yield: 3 Servings
Total Time: 25 Minutes
Prep Time: 15 Minutes
Cook Time: 10 Minutes

Ingredients
- 3 large zucchinis, julienne
- 1 cup cherry tomatoes, halved
- ½ cup basil
- 2 red onion, thinly sliced
- ¼ teaspoon salt
- 1 teaspoon cayenne pepper
- 2 tablespoons lemon juice

Directions
To create zucchini noodles (zoodles) using a vegetable peeler, shave the zucchini with the peeler lengthwise until you get to the core with the seeds. Turn the zucchini, and repeat the process is creating long strips. Continue repeating the process until you have shaved all the zucchini into strips, and discard the seeds. Now lay your strips on a cutting board, and slice lengthwise to the desired thickness that you would like your zoodle to be.

Tip: Alternately this process could also be done using a spiralizer, mandolin, or julienne peeler.

In a bowl add zucchini, onion, basil, tomatoes, basil and toss to combine. Sprinkle salt and cayenne pepper on top. Drizzle lemon juice. Serve and enjoy.

25. __Roasted Cauliflower__

Yield: 8 Servings
Total Time: 35 Minutes
Prep Time: 5 Minutes
Cook Time: 30 Minutes

Ingredients
- cauliflower (1 large head)
- melted coconut oil (2 tbsp.)
- fresh thyme (2 tbsp.)
- Celtic sea salt (1 tsp.)
- fresh ground pepper (1 tsp.)
- roasted garlic (1 head; optional)

GARNISH:
- burrata cheese (8 oz.' if not dairy sensitive)
- fresh thyme (2 tbsp.)

Directions
Heat oven to 425 degrees. Rinse cauliflower, trim, core, and slice. Lay cauliflower evenly on a rimmed baking tray. Dribble the coconut oil evenly over cauliflower; sprinkle with thyme leaves, a pinch of salt and dash of pepper (if using roasted garlic, squeeze on the cauliflower at this time).

Roast until the cauliflower is slightly caramelized, turning once, about half an hour. Use fresh thyme leaves and burrata cheese to garnish.

Nutritional Information per Serving:
Calories: 129 Total Fat: 11 g; Carbs: 6 g; Dietary Fiber: 3 g; Sugars: 3 g; Protein: 7 g; Cholesterol: 16 mg; Sodium: 471 mg

26. __Keto Garlic Gnocchi__

Yield: 2 Servings
Total Time: 25 Minutes
Prep Time: 20 Minutes
Cook Time: 5 Minutes

Ingredients
- Kraft Low-Moisture Part-Skim mozzarella (2 cups shredded. If this particular cheese is not used, it will fall apart when boiling.)
- egg yolks (3)
- granulated garlic (1 tsp.)
- butter & olive oil for sautéing

Directions
Combine cheese and garlic in a microwavable bowl. Use the microwave to melt cheese. Give it a time period of 1-1 ½ mins. Fold in egg yolks individually until a consistent dough is formed (this actually takes some effort). Divide dough into 4 balls. Put to chill in the refrigerator for not less than 10 mins.

Grease your hands and a piece of parchment paper lightly and roll each ball into a 15" log. Slice log into 1" pieces (gnocchi). Boil half a gallon of water in a large pot. Put all the gnocchi into the pot and cook until they are afloat. This takes about 3 mins. Use a colander to strain off liquid.

On medium high flame, heat a suitable size non-stick pan. Pour a tablespoon of olive oil in the pan and add a tablespoon of butter. Place gnocchi in the pan and sauté each side until golden brown. Add salt and pepper to taste. Serve!

Nutritional Information per Serving:
Calories: 244; Total Fat: 7 g; Carbs: 5.3 g; Dietary Fiber: 2.1 g; Sugars: 6.1 g; Protein: 40 g; Cholesterol: 297 mg; Sodium: 852 mg

CHAPTER 5: Dinner Recipes

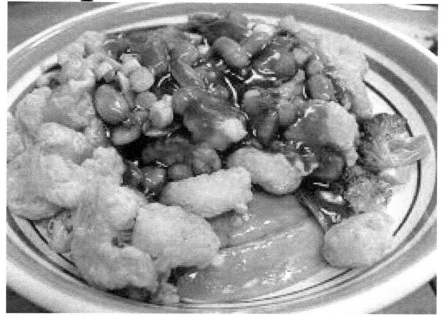

Thank you for allowing us to expose you to the large variety of Keto Vegetarian recipes that you can enjoy, please feel free to leave us a positive review if you like what you are about to read through.

27. Crepe Fettuccine with Tomatoes, Fresh Mozzarella and Pesto

Yield: 6-8 Servings
Total Time: 1 Hour and 50 Minutes
Prep Time: 20 Minutes

Cook Time: 1 Hour and 30 Minutes

Ingredients
- all-purpose ricotta crepes (15, see recipe)
- olive oil (2 tbsp.)
- assorted fresh cherry tomatoes (1 lb., cut into halves and quarters)
- red chili flakes (1/2 tsp., crushed)
- fresh mozzarella (1 lb., removed from the water and cubed)
- parmesan cheese (1/4 cup cheese, grated)
- fresh basil (16 leaves)
- pesto sauce (1 tbsp)
- salt and fresh cracked pepper, to taste

Directions
Put the crepes in small stacks of 5; roll them into little tight logs. Slice crepe into ½" sizes. You can go thinner or fatter as desired. After cutting, fluff the crepe noodles into a neat little pile. Put aside.

Heat oil in a suitable size sauté pan, on medium flame. When hot, add assorted tomatoes, chili flakes and a pinch of pepper and salt. Sauté for 60 secs. Add in pesto and noodles and mix until well coated. Cook for 60 secs.

Stir in mozzarella and cook until the cheese starts melting. Add the fresh mozzarella and toss. Shared in 4 portions. Use fresh basil and parmesan cheese to garnish. Serve!

Nutritional Information per Serving:
Calories: 654; Total Fat: 34 g; Carbs: 29 g; Dietary Fiber: 5 g; Sugars: 18 g; Protein: 61 g; Cholesterol: 124 mg; Sodium: 1096 mg

28. <u>Pasta and Pepper Primavera</u>

Yield: 4 Servings
Total Time: 18 Minutes
Prep Time: 3 Minutes
Cook Time: 15 Minutes

Ingredients
- Spaghetti (4 oz, uncooked)
- Garlic (2 teaspoons, diced)
- Lemon peel (1/2 teaspoon, shredded)
- Thyme (1/2 teaspoon, crushed)
- Black pepper (1/4 teaspoon)
- Butter (1 tablespoon)
- Olive oil (1 tablespoon)
- Frozen peppers and onions (16 oz)
- White wine (1/4 cup, dry)
- Lemon juice (1 tablespoon)
- Salt (1/4 teaspoon)
- Red pepper (1/4 teaspoon, crushed)
- Parmesan cheese (1 oz, shaved)

Directions
Cook pasta as directed on package, drain and put aside. Heat oil in a skillet and sauté garlic for 1minute. Add frozen peppers and cook for 2 minutes. Add wine, thyme, black pepper, lemon juice, red pepper and salt to skillet. Stir to combine, bring to a boil and cook for 4 minutes until vegetables are tender. Remove from flame and add butter.

Add reserved pasta to vegetables and toss. Serve pasta topped with lemon peel and Parmesan cheese.

Nutritional Information per Serving:
Calories: 371.7; Total Fat: 12 g; Carbs: 55 g; Dietary Fiber: 13.2 g; Sugars: 2.9 g; Protein: 18.6 g; Cholesterol: 9.9 mg; Sodium: 462.6 mg

29. <u>Low Carb Mushroom Risotto</u>

Yield: 4 Servings
Prep Time: 5 Minutes
Cook Time: 10 Minutes
Total Time: 15 Minutes

Ingredients
- cauliflower (4 ½ cups, "riced")
- coconut oil (3 tbsp., divided)
- Portobello mushrooms (1 lb., thinly sliced)
- white mushrooms (1 lb., thinly sliced)
- 2 shallots (2, diced)
- cup organic veggie broth (1/4 cup)
- Celtic sea salt (to taste)
- freshly ground black pepper (to taste)
- finely chopped chives (3 tbsp., finely chopped)
- butter (4 tbsp.)
- parmesan cheese (½ cup, freshly grated)

Directions

Use a food processor or a cheese grater to pulse cauliflower florets until they resemble small grains of rice. In a large saucepan, heat 2 tbsp. of oil over medium-high flame. Add the mushrooms and sauté for 3 mins., until mushrooms are tender. Clear saucepan of mushroom and liquid and put aside.

Add remaining 1 tbsp. of oil to skillet; toss shallots and cook in 60 secs. Stir in cauliflower rice, stir for 2 mins. until coated with oil. Add broth to the riced cauliflower and stir until totally absorbed. This takes about 5 mins. Remove pot from heat, mix in mushrooms with liquid, chives butter, and parmesan cheese. Add salt and pepper to taste.

Nutritional Information per Serving:
Calories: 438; Total Fat: 17.1 g; Carbs: 57 g; Dietary Fiber: 3 g; Sugars: 8 g; Protein: 12 g; Cholesterol: 56 mg; Sodium: 221 mg

30. <u>**Keto Vegan "Zoodles"**</u>

Yield: 4 Servings
Total Time: 30 Minutes
Prep Time: 5 Minutes
Cook Time: 25 Minutes

Ingredients
- zucchini (4 medium, use a julienne or vegetable peeler to slice)
- avocado Pesto (1/2 cup))
- avocados (2, average))
- olives (1 cup, pitted)
- sun-dried tomatoes (1/4 cup, sun-dried, drained)
- fresh basil (1/4 cup)
- extra virgin coconut oil (2 tbsp.)
- salt (1/4 tsp.)

Directions
Create zucchini noodles by using a spiralizer. Remove the soft core of the zucchini, chop it and add to the zoodles (spiralized zucchini). Use coconut oil to grease a large saucepan. Place zoodles in a saucepan and cook for a brief period of 2-5 mins. The accuracy of the time depends on how soon you want the zoodles.

Peel the avocados and cut them into halves. Take out the seed and cut into thin pegs. Strain olives and sun-dried tomatoes. Chop tomatoes after straining. Spoon in pesto as soon as zoodles are removed from heat. Mix until thoroughly combined. Add salt to taste. Transfer to a serving plate and arrange olives, tomatoes, fresh basil, and avocado. Enjoy!

Nutritional Information per Serving:
Calories: 449; Total Fat: 42 g; Carbs: 20 g; Dietary Fiber: 11.4 g; Sugars: 2 g; Protein: 6.3 g; Cholesterol: 0 mg; Sodium: 409 mg

31. Whiskey-Ginger Grilled Tofu

Yield: 4 Servings
Total Time: 1 Hour 10 Minutes
Prep Time: 10 Minutes
Cook Time: 1 Hour

Ingredients
- Coconut Aminos (1/3 cup)
- Lime Juice (2 tablespoons)
- Ginger (2 teaspoons, grated)
- Red Pepper (1/4 teaspoon, minced)
- Olive Oil cooking spray
- Cornstarch (1/2 teaspoon)
- Stevia (3 tablespoons)
- Sesame Oil (2 teaspoons)
- Garlic (2 cloves, crushed)
- Water (1 tablespoon)
- Sesame Seeds (1 teaspoon, toasted)
- Tofu (12 ounces extra firm, drained, sliced)
- Whiskey (1/3 cup)

Directions
Cut your tofu about 1/2-inch-thick squares. Next mix whiskey, soy sauce, hoisin sauce, lime juice, ginger, red pepper, brown sugar, sesame oil, and garlic. Place the tofu in a Ziploc bag and pour the marinade on the stripes. Leave refrigerated for one hour. Warm up the grill and remove the marinade meat from the refrigerator.

Spray the cooking spray on the grill, place tofu on the hot grill and allow each strip to be grilled for about five minutes. Boil water, cornstarch, and the marinade mix leave to simmer for 10 minutes. Pour the mixture over the tofu strips and sprinkle sesame seeds. Serve & Enjoy!

Nutritional Information per Serving:
Calories: 193; Total Fat: 11.8 g; Carbs: 7.1 g; Dietary Fiber: 2.2 g; Sugars: 3.2 g; Protein: 1.1 g; Cholesterol: 9.9 mg; Sodium: 665 mg

32. <u>Beer Battered Coconut Tofu</u>

Yield: 11 Servings
Total Time: 1 Hour 40 Minutes
Prep Time: 10 Minutes
Cook Time: 1 Hour 30 Minutes

Ingredients
Protein
- Tofu (2½ lb., extra firm, drained, largely sliced)

Batter
- Eggs (2)
- Beer (100ml)
- Hot Sauce (4tsp.)
- Garlic (12g, chopped)

Coconut & Spice Mix
- White Pepper (1 tsp)
- Black Pepper (1 tsp.)
- Salt (2 tsp.)
- Dried Coconut (2 cups, grated)

General
- Coconut Oil (1L)

Directions
Set tofu to marinate for at least 30 minutes in the batter. Heat oil in a large skillet, over medium heat. Combine the coconut and spices together. Roll the tofu pieces into your coconut mixture so that they are evenly coated, then dip the pieces into your batter and back into the coconut. Once coated, carefully place your tofu pieces in the heated oil (the tofu should be completely covered in oil). Allow cooking until evenly golden brown in appearance. Drain excess oil on a paper towel then serve.

Nutritional Information per Serving:
Calories: 511; Total Fat: 31.6 g; Carbs: 43.7 g; Dietary Fiber: 2.8 g; Sugars: 3.5 g; Protein: 11.6 g; Cholesterol: 0 mg; Sodium: 665 mg

33. <u>Low Carb Cauliflower and Macaroni Cheese</u>

Yield: 4 Servings
Total Time: 1 Hour
Prep Time: 15 Minutes
Cook Time: 45 Minutes

Ingredients
- cauliflower florets (5 cups)
- sea salt and pepper to taste
- coconut milk (1 cup, canned)
- homemade broth (1/2 cup)
- coconut flour (2 tbsp., sifted)
- soy free organic egg (1, beaten)
- grass-fed cheddar cheese (2 cups)

Directions
Heat oven to 350 degrees F. Add some salt to the cauliflower, steam until firm. Place the florets in a properly greased oven proof dish. Heat coconut milk with desired salt and pepper using medium heat. Stir in broth. Add coconut flour to the mixture, stir. Cook until sauce starts bubbling.

Take sauce from heat and incorporate the egg. When sauce becomes thicken, pour it over cauliflower. Mix in cheese and bake for a 35 – 40 min. period. At the last 5 mins. set the oven gauge to broil; this will give the mac and cheese a great color on the top.

Nutritional Information per Serving:
Calories: 229; Total Fat: 14 g; Carbs: 11 g; Dietary Fiber: 1 g; Sugars: 2 g; Protein: 15 g; Cholesterol: 43 mg; Sodium: 250 mg

34. <u>Smoked Tofu Quesadillas</u>

Yield: 4 Servings
Total Time: 30 Minutes
Prep Time: 10 Minutes
Cook Time: 20 Minutes

Ingredients
- Tofu (1lb, extra firm, drained, thinly sliced, smoked, grilled)
- Paleo Tortillas (12)
- Coconut oil (2 tablespoons)
- Jalapeño (4, chopped)
- Cheddar cheese (6 slices)
- Sundried tomatoes (2 tablespoons)
- Cilantro (1 tablespoon)
- Sour cream (5 tablespoons)

Directions
Lay one tortilla flat and fill with tofu, tomato, jalapeno, cheese and top with oil. Repeat for as many as you need. Bake for 5 minutes and remove from flame. Top with sour cream and enjoy!

Nutritional Information per Serving:
Calories: 511; Total Fat: 31.6 g; Carbs: 43.7 g; Dietary Fiber: 2.8 g; Sugars: 3.5 g; Protein: 11.6 g; Cholesterol: 0 mg; Sodium: 665 mg

35. <u>Tofu with Chive Sauce</u>

Yield: 4 Servings
Total Time: 30 Minutes
Prep Time: 10 Minutes
Cook Time: 20 Minutes

Ingredients

- Tofu (1lb, extra firm, drained, cut into halves)
- Black pepper (1/4 teaspoon)
- Olive oil (1 tablespoon)
- White wine (1/2 cup, dry)
- Chives (1 tablespoon, snipped)
- Salt (1/4 teaspoon)
- Almond flour (3 tablespoons)
- Shallots (1/2 cup, diced)
- Tofu stock (1 cup)

Directions

Use pepper and salt to season tofu. Put flour into a dish and use to coat tofu thoroughly. Next heat oil in a skillet and cook for 5 minutes on one side until golden. Flip tofu and cook for 5 minutes on the other side; remove from heat and put aside.

Prepare sauce by heating a skillet and cooking shallots for 2 minutes then add wine and cook for 1 minute until wine reduces by half. Use a spoon to scrape pan. Add broth to skillet and cook for 4 minutes, stir and cook until liquid reduces by half. Add chives and then add tofu. Heat thoroughly and serve.

Nutritional Information per Serving:

Calories: 189.1; Total Fat: 10.3 g; Carbs: 9.2 g; Dietary Fiber: 0.6 g; Sugars: 3.7 g; Protein: 15.9 g; Cholesterol: 0 mg; Sodium: 302.7 mg

36. __Asian-Inspired Tofu__

Yield: 8 Servings
Total Time: 1 Hour 15 Minutes
Prep Time: 15 Minutes
Cook Time: 1 Hour

Ingredients:

- Tofu (3 lbs., cubed)
- Extra Virgin Coconut Oil (2 tbsp.)
- Garlic (4 cloves, chopped)
- Ginger (2 tbsp., chopped)
- Anise Seed (1 tsp)
- Fennel Seed (1 tsp)
- Coconut Amino (1/2 cup)
- Stevia (2 tbsp.)
- Apple Cider Vinegar (2 tbsp.)
- Fish Sauce (1 tbsp.)
- Sesame Oil (2 tbsp.)
- Sesame Seeds (1 tbsp.)

Directions

Put tofu into a large bowl, drain or pat to dry. In a small saucepan heat oil then add garlic, ginger, fennel seed and anise and cook for 3 minutes. Add stevia, vinegar, amino and fish sauce and cook for a minute. Remove from flame and add sesame oil. Pour mixture over tofu and stir. Cool and refrigerate overnight, you may occasionally stir as it marinates. Remove tofu from marinade and bake tofu at 375 °until they are done (about 7 – 10 minutes). Remove from heat, sprinkle with sesame seeds and enjoy. Add your favorite side dish or have as is.

Nutritional Information per Serving:
Calories: 305; Total Fat: 20 g; Carbs: 22.75 g; Dietary Fiber: 3.1 g; Sugars: 0.7 g; Protein: 13 g; Cholesterol: 0 mg; Sodium: 175 mg

37. Crispy Vegan Oven Fried Tofu

Yield: 4 Servings
Total Time: 1 Hour 45 Minutes
Prep Time: 15 Minutes
Cook Time: 1 Hour 30 Minutes

Ingredients
- Tofu (1 lb., extra firm, drained, sliced)
- Olive Oil (2 tbsp.)
- Panko Breadcrumbs (1 cup)
- Nutritional Yeast (1 tbsp.)
- Onion Powder (1/2 tsp.)
- Garlic Powder (1/2 tsp.)
- Oregano (1/2 tsp.)
- Salt (1/4 tsp.)

Directions

Combine all the ingredients, except tofu and olive oil in a shallow bowl, and mix well. Set your oven to preheat to 400 degrees F. In a wide bowl combine all your panko crust ingredients.

Brush your tofu pieces with olive oil then dip it into your panko mix so that it's evenly coated, then onto a lined baking sheet. Place into your preheated oven and allow to cook until golden brown in appearance (about 20 – 30 minutes flipping them at half way). Drain excess oil, if any, then serve.

Nutritional Information per Serving:
Calories: 282.3; Total Fat: 20.7 g; Carbs: 13.8 g; Dietary Fiber: 0.7 g; Sugars: 4 g; Protein: 12.3 g; Cholesterol: 0 mg; Sodium: 150 mg

38. <u>Coconut & Almond Crusted Fried Tofu</u>

Yield: 4 Servings
Total Time: 1 Hour 15 Minutes
Prep Time: 15 Minutes
Cook Time: 1 Hour

Ingredients:
- Tofu (1 lb., extra firm, drained, sliced)
- Salt (1/2 tsp.)
- Pepper (1/4 tsp.)
- Almonds (3/4 cup, grated)
- Garlic Powder (1/2 tsp.)
- Chili Powder (1/2 tsp.)
- Eggs (2, beaten)
- Coconut (1/2 cup, grated)
- Vegetable Oil (2 quarts., for frying)

Directions

Heat oil in a large skillet, over medium heat. Season your tofu with the powder spices listed, then roll the tofu pieces in your almonds, then eggs, then coconut so that they are evenly coated.

Once coated, carefully place your tofu pieces in the heated oil (about 3 or 4 at a time, depending on the size of your skillet), Allow to cook until golden brown in appearance. Drain excess oil on a paper towel then serve.

Nutritional Information per Serving:
Calories: 254.3; Total Fat: 24.7 g; Carbs: 5.2 g; Dietary Fiber: 1.5 g; Sugars: 0.4 g; Protein: 6.7 g; Cholesterol: 0 mg; Sodium: 256 mg

39. **<u>Barbe - Fried Tofu</u>**

Yield: 8 Servings
Total Time: 1 Hour 15 Minutes
Prep Time: 15 Minutes
Cook Time: 1 Hour

Ingredients:
- Tofu (2 lbs., extra firm, drained, cubed)
- Salt (2 tsp., to taste)
- Pepper (1 tsp., to taste)
- BBQ Sauce (½ cup, for coating)
- Sesame Seeds (1 tbsp., for garnish)
- Vegetable Oil (2 quarts., for frying)

Directions
Drain your tofu, and wrap in a clean towel. Lay your wrapped tofu on a flat surface, and top with a heavy pan for about 10 minutes. Unwrap, and cut your tofu into cubes. Season your tofu to taste, then roll the tofu pieces in your bbq sauce so that they are evenly coated.

Heat oil in a large skillet, over medium heat. Carefully place your tofu pieces in the heated oil. Allow cooking until golden brown in appearance. Drain excess oil on a paper towel then serve.

Nutritional Information per Serving:
Calories: 207.7; Total Fat: 11.6 g; Carbs: 14.1 g; Dietary Fiber: 2.6 g; Sugars: 7.3 g; Protein: 14.4 g; Cholesterol: 0 mg; Sodium: 356 mg

40. <u>Southern Fried Tofu</u>

Yield: 4 Servings
Total Time: 45 Minutes + Marinating time
Prep Time: 15 Minutes + Marinating time
Cook Time: 30 Minutes

Ingredients
<u>Protein & Marinade</u>
- Tofu (2 lbs., extra firm, cubed)
- Salt (1 teaspoon)
- Cajun Spice (1 teaspoon)
- Rosemary (1/4 teaspoon dried)
- Thyme (1/4 teaspoon ground)
- Sage (1/8 teaspoon, dried)
- Black Pepper (1/8 teaspoon)
- Cayenne Pepper (1/4 teaspoon)
- Buttermilk (2 cups)

<u>Seasoned Flour</u>
- Almond Flour (2 cups)
- Salt (1 teaspoon)
- Paprika (1/2 teaspoon)
- Cayenne Pepper (1/2 teaspoon)
- Garlic Powder (1/2 teaspoon)
- White Pepper (1/2 teaspoon)
- Onion Powder (1/2 teaspoon)
- Coconut Oil (2 ½ quarts., for frying)

Directions

Heat oil in a large skillet, over medium heat. Season your tofu using the protein ingredients and set in the refrigerator to marinate for at least 6 hours. Combine the flour with listed spices then roll the tofu pieces in your flour so that they are evenly coated. Once coated, carefully place your tofu pieces in the heated oil. Allow cooking until golden brown in appearance. Drain excess oil on a paper towel then serve.

Nutritional Information per Serving:
Calories: 341; Total Fat: 22 g; Carbs: 26.2 g; Dietary Fiber: 2.5 g; Sugars: 0.6 g; Protein: 14.7 g; Cholesterol: 0 mg; Sodium: 394 mg

41. <u>Tex Mex White Egg Pizza</u>

Yield: 1 Servings
Total Time: 17 Minutes
Prep Time: 5 Minutes
Cook Time: 12 Minutes

Ingredients
- extra virgin olive oil (2 tbsp.)
- eggs (2 large)
- ground cumin
- kosher salt
- freshly ground black pepper
- filtered water (1 tbsp.)
- Alfredo sauce (⅛ cup)
- jalapeno (½ pickled, minced)
- Monterey jack cheese (1 oz., shredded)
- green/purple onion (1 tbsp. chopped coarsely)

Directions
Heat oven to 350 degrees F. Place extra virgin olive oil in a skillet over medium high heat. Use a spatula to ensure oil also moistens the sides of the skillet. Use kosher salt, cumin, and black pepper to season eggs. Add filtered water and use a fork or whisk to beat until frothy.

Transfer eggs to a heavy ovenproof skillet; cook over the medium high flame and do not stir, until eggs are set at the bottom. The top of the eggs will still be moist and shaky. Not to worry! Use half of the minced pickled jalapeno mixed with Egg Fast Alfredo to top eggs. Add diced green/ purple onion and 1 oz. shredded cheese.

Place pan on the top rack of preheated oven and bake for 4-5 minutes. Switch oven gauge to broil and allow to get bubbly for about 2 minutes or until the cheese, and the sauce is in golden spots. Allow to stand for 5 minutes. Serve and enjoy!

Nutritional Information per Serving:
Calories: 591; Total Fat: 55 g; Carbs: 2 g; Dietary Fiber: 0.2 g; Sugars: 1.3 g; Protein: 22g; Cholesterol: 464 mg; Sodium: 356 mg

42. <u>Grilled Portabella Mushrooms with Canadian Brie</u>

Yield: 1 Servings
Total Time: 20 Minutes
Prep Time: 5 Minutes
Cook Time: 15 Minutes

Ingredients

- Butter (2 tablespoons, melted)
- Garlic (3 cloves, chopped)
- Canadian brie (6 oz., sliced)
- Balsamic vinegar (2 tablespoons)
- Portobello mushrooms (4)
- Salt (1/4 tsp.)
- Baby arugula (1 cup)
- Black pepper (1/4 tsp.)

Directions

Set oven to 450°F or heat grill. Take stems from mushrooms, and thoroughly clean. Combine butter, garlic, and vinegar in a bowl and use to coat mushrooms. Sprinkle with salt and toss.

Put mushrooms on the hollow side facing down into baking dish or on the grill and cook for 3 minutes then flip, add cheese and cook for an additional 3 minutes. Remove from heat and serve topped with arugula. You may also add a splash of vinegar.

Nutritional Information per Serving:
Calories: 233; Total Fat: 19 g; Carbs: 6 g; Dietary Fiber: 1.2 g; Sugars: 1.3 g; Protein: 11 g; Cholesterol: 0 mg; Sodium: 334 mg

43. <u>Keto Vegetable Wrap</u>

Yield: 1 Servings
Total Time: 20 Minutes
Prep Time: 5 Minutes
Cook Time: 15 Minutes

Ingredients
- Vegetable oil (2 tablespoons)]
- Onion (1/2 cup, chopped)
- Thai red curry (1 cup)
- Wonton wrappers (1 dozen)
- Canned carrots (3 cups)
- Flour (1/4 cup, just for dusting)
- Oil (quart)

Directions
Heat oil in a large skillet and put in the onion. Cook for 15 minutes, stirring frequently. Put in carrots along with curry and cook for 5 minutes. Use flour to dust baking sheet and slice wrappers across to form triangles.

Put 1 tablespoon carrots into the wrapper and wet edges with water, top with another wrapper and press to seal. Place on baking sheet. Repeat until all wrappers are used. Heat quart oil in a pot and fry a few samosas at a time until golden. Serve with your desired chutney.

Nutritional Information per Serving:
Calories: 265.4; Total Fat: 6.7 g; Carbs: 46 g; Dietary Fiber: 10 g; Sugars: 5.9 g; Protein: 10 g; Cholesterol: 0 mg; Sodium: 400 mg

44. **<u>Nuevo Leon Tamales</u>**

Yield: 16 Servings
Total Time: 1 hour 20 minutes
Prep Time: 10 Minutes
Cook Time: 1 hour 10 minutes

Ingredients:
- 1 lb. portabella mushrooms
- 1 garlic clove, minced
- 1 teaspoon stevia
- 2 tablespoons olive oil
- 4 tablespoons chopped green olives
- ¼ teaspoon ground cumin
- 5 whole dried chilies
- 16 corn husks, soaked in water for at least 30 minutes

<u>For the dough:</u>
- 2 cups masa harina
- 1 ¼ cup vegetable broth
- ½ teaspoon baking powder
- ½ teaspoon garlic powder
- ½ teaspoon salt
- 2 tablespoons butter, melted

Directions:
Prepare the dough. In a bowl combine the dough ingredients. Mix with clean hands until you have a smooth dough. Place aside. Prepare the filling: separate the portabella stems and caps. Cook the stems in 2 cups water and a pinch of salt until tender. Heat olive oil in a small pan. Add the sliced portabella caps and cook until soft and tender.

Drain the stems and chop finely. Combine with caps. Soak the chilies in warm water for 15 minutes. Place in a food blender with cumin and olives. Process until smooth. Combine the prepared sauce with mushrooms and cook for 2 minutes. Drain and pat dry the corn husks. Spread around 3 tablespoons prepared dough down the husk, leaving 1-inch border free.

Spoon 2 tablespoons prepare mushroom filling down the center of the dough. Wrap the dough around filling then fold the sides of the husk wrapping all around the filling. Fold up the narrow end of husk and repeat the process with remaining. Place the tamales in a steaming basket and steam for 50 minutes. Serve while still hot.

Nutritional Information per Serving:
Calories: 142; Total Fat: 4.3 g; Carbs: 25 g; Dietary Fiber: 4 g; Sugars: 1.2 g; Protein: 5 g; Cholesterol: 8 mg; Sodium: 189 mg

45. **Sesame Zucchini Zoodles**

Yield: 3 Servings
Total Time: 25 Minutes
Prep Time:10 Minutes
Cook Time: 15 Minutes

Ingredients:
- 3 medium zucchinis
- ½ cup sesame seeds
- ¼ teaspoon garlic paste
- 3 tablespoons sesame oil
- 1 carrot, shredded
- ½ teaspoon white pepper
- ¼ teaspoon salt

Directions
To create zucchini noodles (zoodles) using a vegetable peeler, shave the zucchini with the peeler lengthwise until you get to the core with the seeds. Turn the zucchini, and repeat the process is creating long strips. Continue repeating the process until you have shaved all the zucchini into strips, and discard the seeds. Now lay your strips on a cutting board, and slice lengthwise to the desired thickness that you would like your zoodle to be.

Tip: Alternately this process could also be done using a spiralizer, mandolin, or julienne peeler.

Heat oil in a pan and add garlic, stir for 30 seconds. Add zucchini and mix thoroughly. Cook for 10-15 minutes on medium heat. Sprinkle sesame seeds and mix to combine.
Season with pepper and salt. Transfer to serving the dish and place shredded carrot on top. Serve and enjoy.

Nutritional Information per Serving:
Calories: 290; Total Fat: 29 g; Carbs: 6 g; Dietary Fiber: 4 g; Sugars: 1 g; Protein: 6 g; Cholesterol: 0 mg; Sodium: 220 mg

46. __Zoodles with Sesame Spinach__

Yield: 2 Servings
Total Time: 20 Minutes
Prep Time: 10 Minutes
Cook Time: 10 Minutes

Ingredients
- 1 cup baby spinach
- 1 cup sesame seeds
- 2 tablespoons lime juice
- 2 large zucchinis, julienne
- 2 tablespoons olive oil
- 2-3 garlic cloves, minced
- 1 tablespoon fish sauce
- 2 tablespoons tamari sauce
- ¼ teaspoon salt
- 1 cup green onion, chopped

Directions
To create zucchini noodles (zoodles) using a vegetable peeler, shave the zucchini with the peeler lengthwise until you get to the core with the seeds. Turn the zucchini, and repeat the process is creating long strips. Continue repeating the process until you have shaved all the zucchini into strips, and discard the seeds. Now lay your strips on a cutting board, and slice lengthwise to the desired thickness that you would like your zoodle to be.
Tip: Alternately this process could also be done using a spiralizer, mandolin, or julienne peeler.
Heat oil in pan and fry garlic for 30 seconds. Add in zucchini with spinach and stir for 3-4 minutes on high heat. Season with salt, sesame seeds, fish sauce, tamari sauce, and cook for another 4-5 minutes on low flame. Transfer to serving bowl top with green onion and drizzle lemon juice. Enjoy.

Nutritional Information per Serving:

Calories: 591; Total Fat: 50 g; Carbs: 28 g; Dietary Fiber: 11.5 g; Sugars: 3 g; Protein: 18 g; Cholesterol: 0 mg; Sodium: 1155 mg

47. <u>Squash tamales</u>

Yield: 30 Tamales
Total Time: 40 Minutes
Prep Time:15 Minutes
Cook Time: 2 Hours

Ingredients:

- 4 ½ cups masa harina
- 1 teaspoon baking powder
- 1 teaspoon garlic powder
- 2 tablespoons lime juice
- 1 teaspoon ground cumin
- 1 teaspoon sweet paprika
- 2 ¾ cups vegetable broth

<u>The filling</u>:

- 1 ½ cups diced Kabocha squash
- 4 tablespoons sunflower oil
- ½ onion, diced small
- 1 ½ cups crumbled tempeh
- 1 teaspoon ground cumin
- 3 cups stemmed and chopped kale
- ½ teaspoon red pepper flakes
- ½ teaspoon cayenne pepper
- ½ teaspoon smoked paprika
- 30 corn husks, soaked in water for at least 30 minutes

Directions:

Prepare the dough: In a bowl combine first seven ingredients. Stir in clean hands and place aside. Meanwhile, heat the oil in a skillet. Add the onions and cook for 4 minutes.

Add the tempeh and squash and cook for 5-6 minutes. Lower the heat and add the remaining filling ingredients. Give it all a good stir and cook for 4 minutes or until kale is wilted. Place aside to cool.

Drain and pat dry the corn husks. Spread around ¼ cup prepared dough down the husk, leaving 1-inch border free. Spoon 3 tablespoons prepared filling down the center of the dough. Wrap the dough around filling then fold the sides of the husk wrapping all around the filling. Fold up the narrow end of husk and repeat the process with remaining.

Place the tamales in a steaming basket and steam for 90 minutes.

Best served with tomatillo salsa.

Nutritional Information per Serving:

Calories: 73; Total Fat: 3.2 g; Carbs: 9.2 g; Dietary Fiber: 1 g; Sugars: 1 g; Protein: 3 g; Cholesterol: 0 mg; Sodium: 154 mg

48. Garlicky Parmesan Zoodles

Yield: 2 Servings
Total Time: 20 Minutes
Prep Time:10 Minutes
Cook Time: 10 Minutes

Ingredients
- 3 medium zucchinis
- 1 cup parmesan cheese, shredded
- 1 teaspoon garlic powder
- 2 tablespoons butter
- ½ teaspoon white pepper
- ¼ teaspoon salt

Directions
To create zucchini noodles (zoodles) using a vegetable peeler, shave the zucchini with the peeler lengthwise until you get to the core with the seeds. Turn the zucchini, and repeat the process is creating long strips. Continue repeating the process until you have shaved all the zucchini into strips, and discard the seeds. Now lay your strips on a cutting board, and slice lengthwise to the desired thickness that you would like your zoodle to be.

Tip: Alternately this process could also be done using a spiralizer, mandolin, or julienne peeler.

Melt butter in a pan and sauté zucchini for 1-2 minutes. Sprinkle garlic powder, and cover with lid, cook on low heat for 5 minutes. Add parmesan cheese and stir thoroughly. Sprinkle salt and pepper. Serve and enjoy.

Nutritional Information per Serving:
Calories: 363; Total Fat: 26 g; Carbs: 15 g; Dietary Fiber: 2.6 g; Sugars: 0 g; Protein: 20 g; Cholesterol: 74 mg; Sodium: 1291 mg

49. <u>CHAPTER 6: Slow Cooker Recipes</u>

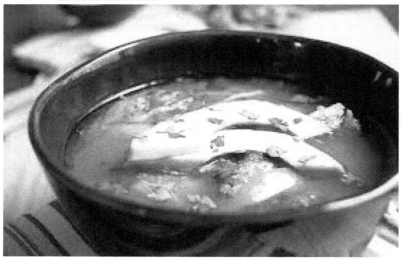

Thank you for allowing us to expose you to the large variety of Keto Vegetarian recipes that you can enjoy, please feel free to leave us a positive review if you like what you are about to read through.

50. <u>Avocado Basil Pesto Zoodles</u>

Yield: 4 Servings
Total Time: 4 Hours 10 Minutes
Prep Time:10 Minutes
Cook Time: 4 hours

Ingredients
- 5 medium zucchinis
- 3 avocadoes, pitted, pulp
- ½ cup basil leaves

- 2 tablespoons coconut oil
- 2-3 garlic cloves, minced
- ½ teaspoon white pepper
- ¼ teaspoon salt
- 2 tablespoon lemon juice
- 4-5 cherry tomatoes halved

Directions

To create zucchini noodles (zoodles) using a vegetable peeler, shave the zucchini with the peeler lengthwise until you get to the core with the seeds. Turn the zucchini, and repeat the process is creating long strips. Continue repeating the process until you have shaved all the zucchini into strips, and discard the seeds. Now lay your strips on a cutting board, and slice lengthwise to the desired thickness that you would like your zoodle to be.

Tip: Alternately this process could also be done using a spiralizer, mandolin, or julienne peeler.

In a food processor add avocado, basil, salt, pepper, garlic, lemon juice, oil and blend until puree. Transfer to bowl. Now add zoodles in pesto and mix thoroughly. Transfer zoodles into your slow cooker, place cherry tomatoes on top, close the lid, and set to cook on low for about 4 hours. Serve hot.

Nutritional Information per Serving:

Calories: 194; Total Fat: 15.1 g; Carbs: 13.4 g; Dietary Fiber: 7 g; Sugars: 2.4 g; Protein: 7 g; Cholesterol: 0 mg; Sodium: 153 mg

51. <u>Lemon Basil Zoodles</u>

Yield: 2 Servings
Total Time: 4 Hours 10 Minutes
Prep Time:10 Minutes
Cook Time: 4 Hours

Ingredients

- 2 large zucchinis
- 2 tablespoons lemon juice

- 1 tablespoon vinegar
- 2-3 garlic cloves, minced
- ¼ teaspoon salt
- 1 pinch white pepper
- 3-4 basil leaves, chopped
- 1 teaspoon ginger paste
- 2 tablespoons butter

Directions

To create zucchini noodles (zoodles) using a vegetable peeler, shave the zucchini with the peeler lengthwise until you get to the core with the seeds. Turn the zucchini, and repeat the process is creating long strips. Continue repeating the process until you have shaved all the zucchini into strips, and discard the seeds. Now lay your strips on a cutting board, and slice lengthwise to the desired thickness that you would like your zoodle to be.

Tip: Alternately this process could also be done using a spiralizer, mandolin, or julienne peeler.

Melt butter in your slow cooker and sauté ginger with garlic. Add zucchini and basil, stir well. Season with salt and pepper. Pour in vinegar, cover the lid, and cook for 4 hours on low. Transfer to serving platter and drizzle lemon juice. Serve and enjoy.

Nutritional Information per Serving:

Calories: 147; Total Fat: 12.2 g; Carbs: 8 g; Dietary Fiber: 2 g; Sugars: 0.4 g; Protein: 4 g; Cholesterol: 31 mg; Sodium: 388 mg

52. Quick Mushrooms Spinach Sauté with Zucchini Noodles

Yield: 3 Servings
Total Time: 4 Hours 10 Minutes
Prep Time:10 Minutes
Cook Time: 4 Hours

Ingredients
- Organic egg (1)
- Scallions (2 stalks, diced)
- Fresh Shitake Mushrooms (3)
- Tamari Sauce (1 teaspoon)
- Baby spinach (3 handfuls)
- Zucchini (1 large)
- Garlic (3 cloves, chopped)
- Ginger (2 teaspoons, diced)
- Cremini mushrooms (1 handful)
- White pepper (1/2 tsp.)

Directions
To create zucchini noodles (zoodles) using a vegetable peeler, shave the zucchini with the peeler lengthwise until you get to the core with the seeds. Turn the zucchini, and repeat the process is creating long strips. Continue repeating the process until you have shaved all the zucchini into strips, and discard the seeds. Now lay your strips on a cutting board, and slice lengthwise to the desired thickness that you would like your zoodle to be.

Tip: Alternately this process could also be done using a spiralizer, mandolin, or julienne peeler.

Heat skillet and add oil to pan then fry an egg and remove from skillet and set aside. Put 2/3 garlic into the skillet along with scallions; sauté for 1 minute then put in mushrooms.

Season with pepper and tamari sauce and cook until mushrooms are tender. Remove from pot and put aside. Put leftover garlic into the skillet along with ginger. Cook until fragrant then put in spinach and stir fry. Transfer zoodles into your slow cooker, place your remaining ingredients on top, close the lid, and set to cook on low for about 4 hours. Serve hot, topped with an egg.

Nutritional Information per Serving:
Calories: 66; Total Fat: 3.2 g; Carbs: 5.3 g; Dietary Fiber: 1.2 g; Sugars: 0.6 g; Protein: 5 g; Cholesterol: 206 mg; Sodium: 71 mg

53. <u>Avocado Salsa Zoodles</u>

Yield: 2 Servings
Total Time: 4 Hours 15 Minutes
Prep Time: 15 Minutes
Cook Time: 4 Hours

Ingredients
- 2 medium zucchinis
- 1 Hass avocado, pitted, chunks
- ¼ teaspoon salt
- ¼ teaspoon black pepper
- 4 tablespoons lemon juice
- 2 tablespoon apple cider vinegar
- 3 tablespoon stevia
- ½ teaspoon dill, chopped
- Few coriander leaves for garnishing

Directions
To create zucchini noodles (zoodles) using a vegetable peeler, shave the zucchini with the peeler lengthwise until you get to the core with the seeds. Turn the zucchini, and repeat the process is creating long strips. Continue repeating the process until you have shaved all the zucchini into strips, and discard the seeds. Now lay your strips on a cutting board, and slice lengthwise to the desired thickness that you would like your zoodle to be.
Tip: Alternately this process could also be done using a spiralizer, mandolin, or julienne peeler.
Transfer zoodles into your slow cooker, close the lid, and set to cook on low for about 4 hours. Combine avocado, dill, salt, pepper, stevia, vinegar, lemon juice, and mix. Place zoodle in serving platter and top with mango salsa. Garnish with coriander leaves. Serve and enjoy.

Nutritional Information per Serving:
Calories: 257; Total Fat: 16 g; Carbs: 51 g; Dietary Fiber: 10 g;
Sugars: 14 g; Protein: 7 g; Cholesterol: 206 mg; Sodium: 71 mg

54. **Carrot and Beet Zoodles**

Yield: 4 Servings
Total Time: 4 Hours 10 Minutes
Prep Time:10 Minutes
Cook Time: 4 Hours

Ingredients

- 3 large beetroots, julienne
- 2 carrots, peeled, julienne
- 1 apples, peeled, julienne
- 1 tablespoons olive oil
- ¼ teaspoon salt
- ¼ teaspoon black pepper
- 6 tablespoons lemon juice
- 2 tablespoon sunflower seeds
- ½ cup peas shoots, roughly chopped
- 2 tablespoon pine seeds

Directions

To create zucchini noodles (zoodles) using a vegetable peeler, shave the zucchini with the peeler lengthwise until you get to the core with the seeds. Turn the zucchini, and repeat the process is creating long strips. Continue repeating the process until you have shaved all the zucchini into strips, and discard the seeds. Now lay your strips on a cutting board, and slice lengthwise to the desired thickness that you would like your zoodle to be.

Tip: Alternately this process could also be done using a spiralizer, mandolin, or julienne peeler.

Transfer zoodles into your slow cooker, close the lid, and set to cook on low for about 4 hours. Take a large bowl and add all ingredients, toss to combine. Add to serving bowl and serve immediately.

Nutritional Information per Serving:

Calories: 557; Total Fat: 49 g; Carbs: 36 g; Dietary Fiber: 44 g; Sugars: 8 g; Protein: 5 g; Cholesterol: 0 mg; Sodium: 715 mg

55. Beet Fettuccine with Avocado Pesto

Yield: 3 Servings
Total Time: 6 Hours 10 Minutes
Prep Time:10 Minutes
Cook Time: 6 Hours

Ingredients
- 3 large beetroots, fettuccine
- 2 Hass avocadoes pitted
- ¼ cup yogurt
- ½ bunch coriander
- ¼ teaspoon salt
- 1 teaspoon black pepper
- 2 tablespoons lemon juice

Directions
To create beet noodles using a vegetable peeler, shave the beets with the peeler in a circular motion until you get to a point where you can't shave anymore. Continue repeating the process until you have shaved all the beet into strips, and discard the skin. Now lay your strips on a cutting board, and slice lengthwise to the desired thickness that you would like your beet noodle to be.

Tip: Alternately this process could also be done using a spiralizer, mandolin, or julienne peeler.

Transfer beet noodles into your slow cooker, close the lid, and set to cook on low for about 6 hours. In a blender add avocado, coriander, yogurt, salt, pepper, lemon juice and blend until puree. Arrange beetroot fettuccine and top with avocado pesto. Serve and enjoy.

Nutritional Information per Serving:

Calories: 557; Total Fat: 49 g; Carbs: 36 g; Dietary Fiber: 44 g; Sugars: 8 g; Protein: 5 g; Cholesterol: 0 mg; Sodium: 715 mg

56. <u>Beet Zoodles</u>

Yield: 2 Servings
Total Time: 25 Minutes
Prep Time: 15 Minutes
Cook Time: 10 Minutes

Ingredients
- 2 beetroots, peeled, julienne
- 1 tablespoons olive oil
- 1 tablespoon stevia
- 1 teaspoon dill, chopped
- 1 pinch salt

Directions
To create beet noodles using a vegetable peeler, shave the beets with the peeler in a circular motion until you get to a point where you can't shave anymore. Continue repeating the process until you have shaved all the beet into strips, and discard the skin. Now lay your strips on a cutting board, and slice lengthwise to the desired thickness that you would like your beet noodle to be.

Tip: Alternately this process could also be done using a spiralizer, mandolin, or julienne peeler.

Transfer beet noodles into your slow cooker, close the lid, and set to cook on low for about 6 hours. Heat oil in a pan and sauté beetroot for 3-4 minutes. Add stevia, salt and mix well. Add dill and transfer to serving dish. Serve and enjoy.

Nutritional Information per Serving:
Calories: 556; Total Fat: 34 g; Carbs: 28 g; Dietary Fiber: 5 g; Sugars: 6 g; Protein: 49 g; Cholesterol: 325 mg; Sodium: 698 mg

57. Zucchini Zoodles with Strawberry Sauce

Yield: 3 Servings
Total Time: 4 Hours 15 Minutes
Prep Time: 15 Minutes
Cook Time: 4 Hours

Ingredients
- 3 large zucchinis, julienne
- ¼ cup white sesame seeds
- ¼ cup black sesame seeds
- 1 avocado, pitted, sliced
- ¼ teaspoon salt
- ½ teaspoon black pepper
- ½ cup broccoli florets
- 2 cups strawberries
- ½ cup sugar

Directions
To create zucchini noodles (zoodles) using a vegetable peeler, shave the zucchini with the peeler lengthwise until you get to the core with the seeds. Turn the zucchini, and repeat the process is creating long strips. Continue repeating the process until you have shaved all the zucchini into strips, and discard the seeds. Now lay your strips on a cutting board, and slice lengthwise to the desired thickness that you would like your zoodle to be.

Tip: Alternately this process could also be done using a spiralizer, mandolin, or julienne peeler.

Transfer zoodles, sugar, and strawberries into your slow cooker, close the lid, and set to cook on low for about 4 hours. Transfer to blender and blend will puree. Place aside. In a bowl add zucchini zoodles, broccoli, avocado, white sesame seed, black sesame seeds, and toss to combine. Drizzle strawberry sauce on top and serve.

Nutritional Information per Serving:

Calories: 393; Total Fat: 26 g; Carbs: 38 g; Dietary Fiber: 11.2 g; Sugars: 22 g; Protein: 11.2 g; Cholesterol: 0 mg; Sodium: 218 mg

58. Zucchini and Carrot Zoodles with Tomato Sauce

Yield: 2 Servings
Total Time: 3 Hours 15 Minutes
Prep Time: 15 Minutes
Cook Time: 3 Hours

Ingredients

- 2 zucchinis, julienne
- 2 carrots, peeled, julienne
- 1 cup tomatoes, chopped
- 2 tablespoon brown sugar
- ¼ pinch salt
- ¼ cup sun dried tomatoes
- ½ cup cream
- ½ cup water

Directions

To create zucchini noodles (zoodles) using a vegetable peeler, shave the zucchini with the peeler lengthwise until you get to the core with the seeds. Turn the zucchini, and repeat the process is creating long strips. Continue repeating the process until you have shaved all the zucchini into strips, and discard the seeds. Now lay your strips on a cutting board, and slice lengthwise to the desired thickness that you would like your zoodle to be.

Tip: Alternately this process could also be done using a spiralizer, mandolin, or julienne peeler.

In a slow cooker add water, tomatoes, sun dries tomatoes, brown sugar, salt and mix well. Let to cook for 3 hours on low with the lid closed. Add in cream and mix, transfer to a blender and blend well. In platter add carrot and zucchini zoodles and top with tomato sauce.

Enjoy.

Nutritional Information per Serving:
Calories: 225; Total Fat: 13 g; Carbs: 25 g; Dietary Fiber: 5 g;
Sugars: 16 g; Protein: 7 g; Cholesterol: 40 mg; Sodium: 367 mg

59. Creamy Zucchini Zoodles with Brussel Sprouts

Yield: 2 Servings
Total Time: 3 Hours 10 Minutes
Prep Time: 10 Minutes
Cook Time: 3 Hours

Ingredients

- 2 large zucchinis, julienne
- 1 cup sour cream
- 1 cup Brussel sprouts, boiled
- ¼ teaspoon salt
- ¼ teaspoon black pepper
- 2 tablespoons lemon juice
- 2 tablespoons fresh dill, chopped

Directions

To create zucchini noodles (zoodles) using a vegetable peeler, shave the zucchini with the peeler lengthwise until you get to the core with the seeds. Turn the zucchini, and repeat the process is creating long strips. Continue repeating the process until you have shaved all the zucchini into strips, and discard the seeds. Now lay your strips on a cutting board, and slice lengthwise to the desired thickness that you would like your zoodle to be.

Tip: Alternately this process could also be done using a spiralizer, mandolin, or julienne peeler.

Transfer zoodles into your slow cooker with lemon juice, and salt. Cover, and allow to cook on low for 3 hours. In a bowl combine Brussel sprouts with salt, black pepper, lemon juice, and mix well. Add zoodles to a serving platter and top with a puddle of sour cream, Brussel sprouts, and sprinkle dill. Serve and enjoy.

Nutritional Information per Serving:
Calories: 185; Total Fat: 21 g; Carbs: 34 g; Dietary Fiber: 26 g;
Sugars: 16 g; Protein: 78 g; Cholesterol: 357 mg; Sodium: 318 mg

60. Fried Sweet Potato Noodles

Yield: 3 Servings
Total Time: 3 Hours 10 Minutes
Prep Time: 10 Minutes
Cook Time: 3 Hours

Ingredients
- 3 large sweet potatoes, peeled, julienne
- 1 teaspoon thyme
- ½ cup oil, for frying
- ¼ teaspoon salt
- 1 teaspoon cayenne pepper

Directions
To create sweet potato noodles using a vegetable peeler, shave the sweet potato with the peeler lengthwise until you get to the core with the seeds. Turn the sweet potato, and repeat the process is creating long strips. Continue repeating the process until you have shaved all the sweet potato into strips, and discard the seeds. Now lay your strips on a cutting board, and slice lengthwise to the desired thickness that you would like your noodle to be.

Tip: Alternately this process could also be done using a spiralizer, mandolin, or julienne peeler.

Transfer noodles to a slow cooker with 2 tbsp. of water, and set to cook on low for about 3 hours. Heat oil in a pan and deep fry sweet potato noodles. Spread on a paper towel and drain out excess oil. Sprinkle salt and cayenne pepper on top. Serve and enjoy.

Nutritional Information per Serving:
Calories: 236; Total Fat: 17.6 g; Carbs: 16 g; Dietary Fiber: 2 g; Sugars: 3 g; Protein: 5 g; Cholesterol: 5 mg; Sodium: 1318 mg

61. Hot and Spicy Marinara Zucchini

Yield: 4 Servings
Total Time: 4 Hours 10 Minutes
Prep Time: 10 Minutes
Cook Time: 4 Hours

Ingredients
- 3 large zucchinis, julienne
- 1 cup marinara sauce
- ½ cup chili garlic sauce
- 2-3 garlic cloves, minced
- ¼ teaspoon salt
- ¼ teaspoon cayenne pepper
- 1 tablespoon coconut oil

Directions
To create zucchini noodles (zoodles) using a vegetable peeler, shave the zucchini with the peeler lengthwise until you get to the core with the seeds. Turn the zucchini, and repeat the process is creating long strips. Continue repeating the process until you have shaved all the zucchini into strips, and discard the seeds. Now lay your strips on a cutting board, and slice lengthwise to the desired thickness that you would like your zoodle to be.

Tip: Alternately this process could also be done using a spiralizer, mandolin, or julienne peeler.

Transfer noodles to a slow cooker with 2 tbsp. of water, and set to cook on low for about 4 hours. Heat oil in a pan and sauté garlic for 1 minute. Add marinara sauce, chili garlic sauce, salt, and cayenne pepper, toss well. Cook for 3-4 minutes then add zucchini, stir and cook for 5-6 minute. Serve and enjoy.

Nutritional Information per Serving:

Calories: 236; Total Fat: 17.6 g; Carbs: 16 g; Dietary Fiber: 2 g; Sugars: 3 g; Protein: 5 g; Cholesterol: 5 mg; Sodium: 1318 mg

62. __Creamy Cucumber Noodles__

Yield: 2 Servings
Total Time: 4h 10 Minutes
Prep Time: 10 Minutes
Cook Time: 4h Minutes

Ingredients
- 2 large cucumbers, julienne
- 1 cup creamy
- 1 teaspoon garlic powder
- ¼ teaspoon salt
- ¼ teaspoon white pepper

Directions
To create zucchini noodles (noodles) using a vegetable peeler, shave the zucchini with the peeler lengthwise until you get to the core with the seeds. Turn the zucchini, and repeat the process is creating long strips. Continue repeating the process until you have shaved all the zucchini into strips, and discard the seeds. Now lay your strips on a cutting board, and slice lengthwise to the desired thickness that you would like your noodle to be.

__Tip: Alternately this process could also be done using a spiralizer, mandolin, or julienne peeler.__

Transfer noodles to a slow cooker with 2 tbsp. of water, and set to cook on low for about 4 hours. In a medium bowl add all ingredients and toss to combine. Serve and enjoy.

Nutritional Information per Serving:
Calories: 236; Total Fat: 17.6 g; Carbs: 16 g; Dietary Fiber: 2 g; Sugars: 3 g; Protein: 5 g; Cholesterol: 5 mg; Sodium: 1318 mg

63. Gingery Cauliflower Soup

Yield: 4 Servings
Total Time: 8 Hours 15 Minutes
Prep Time: 15 Minutes
Cook Time: 8 Hours

Ingredients
- 1 cup cauliflower florets
- 1 teaspoon ginger paste
- 1 red bell pepper chopped
- 2 cups vegetable broth
- 2 tablespoons vinegar
- 1 lemon, sliced
- 1 green chili, chopped
- 4-5 garlic cloves, minced
- ½ teaspoon black pepper
- ¼ teaspoon salt
- 1 tablespoon oil

Directions
Heat oil in a saucepan, add ginger paste and cook for 1 minute. Cauliflower and fry well for 5-10 minutes. Now add bell pepper, salt, pepper, vinegar, green chilies, lemon slices and mix well.

Remove from heat and add to a slow cooker. Add vegetable broth and leave to cook on low for 8 hours. Spoon into serving bowls. Serve and enjoy.

Nutritional Information per Serving:
Calories: 109; Total Fat: 6 g; Carbs: 11.3 g; Dietary Fiber: 2.6 g; Sugars: 3.7 g; Protein: 5 g; Cholesterol: 4 mg; Sodium: 470 mg

64. Avocado Spinach Pesto Zoodles

Yield: 4 Servings
Total Time: 4 Hours 15 Minutes
Prep Time: 15 Minutes
Cook Time: 4 Hours

Ingredients
- 2 Hass avocadoes
- 1 cup baby spinach
- ½ cup cashews
- 2 tablespoons lime juice
- 1 cup cherry tomatoes, halved
- 2 large zucchinis, julienne
- 2 tablespoons olive oil
- 2-3 garlic cloves, minced
- ½ teaspoon black pepper
- 2 tablespoons tamari sauce
- ¼ teaspoon salt

Directions
To create zucchini noodles (zoodles) using a vegetable peeler, shave the zucchini with the peeler lengthwise until you get to the core with the seeds. Turn the zucchini, and repeat the process is creating long strips. Continue repeating the process until you have shaved all the zucchini into strips, and discard the seeds. Now lay your strips on a cutting board, and slice lengthwise to the desired thickness that you would like your zoodle to be.
Tip: Alternately this process could also be done using a spiralizer, mandolin, or julienne peeler.
Transfer noodles to a slow cooker with 2 tbsp. of water, and set to cook on low for about 4 hours. In a blender add avocado, spinach, salt, pepper, lime juice, cashews, olive oil, and blend well. Top with spinach pesto. Mix to combine. Transfer to serving bowl. Place cherry tomatoes on top. Enjoy.

Nutritional Information per Serving: Calories: 251; Total Fat: 22 g; Carbs: 13 g; Dietary Fiber: 5 g; Sugars: 3 g; Protein: 5 g; Cholesterol: 0 mg; Sodium: 271 mg

65.   Fig and Zoodles

Yield: 2 Servings
Total Time: 4 Hours 10 Minutes
Prep Time: 10 Minutes
Cook Time: 4 Hours

Ingredients

- 1 cup fig, sliced
- 2 large zucchinis, julienne
- ¼ teaspoon white pepper
- 1 tablespoon lime juice
- ¼ teaspoon salt

Directions

To create zucchini noodles (zoodles) using a vegetable peeler, shave the zucchini with the peeler lengthwise until you get to the core with the seeds. Turn the zucchini, and repeat the process is creating long strips. Continue repeating the process until you have shaved all the zucchini into strips, and discard the seeds. Now lay your strips on a cutting board, and slice lengthwise to the desired thickness that you would like your zoodle to be.

Tip: Alternately this process could also be done using a spiralizer, mandolin, or julienne peeler.

Transfer noodles to a slow cooker with 2 tbsp. of water, and set to cook on low for about 4 hours. In a bowl add zucchini, fig and toss to combine. Sprinkle salt and pepper, and drizzle lemon juice. Mix well. Transfer to serving the dish and serve. Enjoy.

Nutritional Information per Serving:
Calories: 192; Total Fat: 1 g; Carbs: 49 g; Dietary Fiber: 19 g;
Sugars: 7.3 g; Protein: 3 g; Cholesterol: 0 mg; Sodium: 299 mg

66. CHAPTER 7: Electric pressure Cooker Recipes

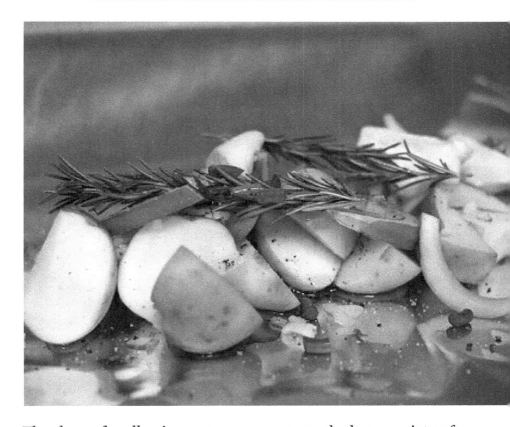

Thank you for allowing us to expose you to the large variety of Keto Vegetarian recipes that you can enjoy, please feel free to leave us a positive review if you like what you are about to read through.

67. Sesame Tofu

Yield: 2 Servings
Total Time: 25 Minutes

Prep Time: 10 Minutes
Cook Time: 15 Minutes

Ingredients
- Tofu (8 oz, dried, diced)
- Oil (2 tablespoons)
- Water (2 tbsp.)
- Black and white sesame seeds (1/2 tsp)
- Scallion (chopped, 1/2 tsp)

Sesame Sauce
- Chinese sesame paste (1/4 tsp)
- Peanut Butter (1 tablespoon)
- Tamari sauce (1 ½ teaspoons)
- Cider Vinegar (1 teaspoon)
- Sesame Oil (1 tablespoon)
- Chili Oil (1/4 tsp)
- Salt (1/4 tsp)
- Coconut sugar (1/4 tsp)

Directions
Set your electric pressure cooker on 'sauté' mode with oil, and allow to heat up. Add tofu and brown on all sides, then set aside to drain. Add all your sauce ingredients then stir in tofu. Close the lid, and switch the cooking modes to 'manual' and set to cook on low pressure for 1 minute.

When the timer goes off perform a quick release, by pressing 'cancel' then carefully turning the pressure valve to venting. **Tip:** Consider using a pot holder, or long spoon to turn the valve as it will be extremely hot. Carefully open, sprinkle with sesame seeds and scallions. Serve and enjoy.

Nutritional Information per Serving:
Calories: 524; Total Fat: 46 g; Carbs: 17.2 g; Dietary Fiber: 5 g; Sugars: 5 g; Protein: 20 g; Cholesterol: 0 mg; Sodium: 459 mg

68. __Cinnamon Almond Flour Muffins__

Yield: 12 Muffins
Total Time: 40 Minutes
Prep Time: 20 Minutes
Cook Time: 20 Minutes

Ingredients:
- Butter (1 tbsp., for greasing)
- Almond Flour (2½ cups + a bit more for dusting)
- Stevia (1/4 cup)
- Baking Powder (2 tsp.)
- Cinnamon (1 tsp., ground)
- Salt (1 tsp., kosher)
- Milk (1 cup, whole)
- Vegetable Oil (1/3 cup)
- Egg (1 large)

Topping
- Butter (4 tbsp., unsalted)
- Almond Flour (1/4 cup)
- Stevia (1/8 cup)
- Salt (1 tsp.)

Directions:
Add all your dry ingredients of the muffin to your electric mixer bowl. In a separate bowl, combine all your muffin's wet ingredients in a separate bowl, then to your dry ingredients and allow to whisk on low until fully combined. Fit your Electric pressure cooker with your steel insert, and a trivet then add your water and set the cooker on the sauté setting to allow it to preheat.

Fill up silicone muffin cups ⅔ way full with your muffin batter and set your muffin cups to set on top of the trivet you fitted into the cooker. Now let's work on your topping. Combine all your topping ingredients into a small bowl and mix with a fork to combine. Crumble the mixture evenly on top of your 12 cups of muffin batter. Prep a cover by cutting a piece of parchment paper and aluminum foil to create a circle then use to cover your muffin cups.

Set your Electric pressure cooker to pressure on high for 8 minutes. Once your timer has finished, press 'cancel' and allow your cooker to cook down naturally for about 15 to 20 minutes before attempting to open. Test your muffins for doneness as you would a cake. Cool, serve, and enjoy!

Nutritional Information per Serving:
Calories: 103.8; Total Fat: 2.5 g; Carbs: 16.7 g; Dietary Fiber: 0.8 g; Sugars: 8.2 g; Protein: 4.3 g; Cholesterol: 93 mg; Sodium: 232.9 mg

69. __Mixed Nuts Cupcakes__

Yields: 12 serving
Total Time: 40 Minutes
Prep Time: 20 Minutes
Cook Time: 20 Minutes

Ingredients
- Coconut Flour (1 ½ cup)
- Baking soda (1 teaspoon)
- Ginger (1 tsp, ground)
- Cinnamon (1 teaspoon)
- Nutmeg (1/4 tsp)
- Salt (1/2 teaspoon)
- Stevia (1/2 cup)
- Coconut Sugar (1/3 cup)
- Baking powder (1/2 teaspoon)
- Olive oil (1/2 cup)
- Greek yogurt (2 teaspoons, vanilla)
- Vanilla (1 teaspoon)
- Almonds (1 cup, crushed)
- Hazelnuts (1/2 cup, crushed)
- Walnuts (1 cup, chopped)

Directions
Sift baking powder, flour, baking soda, cinnamon, ginger, salt and nutmeg in a big bowl. Mix to combine. Whisk oil, coconut sugar, stevia, vanilla, and yogurt together in a different bowl. Add the liquid mixture to dry ingredients and mix to combine; try not to over mix. Put in almonds, walnuts, and hazelnuts and fold in.

Fit your Electric pressure cooker with your steel insert, and a trivet then add your water and set the cooker on the sauté setting to allow it to preheat. Fill up silicone muffin cups ⅔ way full with your cupcake batter and set your muffin cups to set on top of the trivet you fitted into the cooker.

Prep a cover by cutting a piece of parchment paper and aluminum foil to create a circle then use to cover your muffin cups. Set your Electric pressure cooker to pressure on high for 8 minutes.

Once your timer has finished, press 'cancel' and allow your cooker to cook down naturally for about 15 to 20 minutes before attempting to open. Test your cupcakes for doneness as you would a cake. Allow to cool and add the desired frosting.

Nutritional Information per Serving:
Calories: 188.6; Total Fat: 1 g; Carbs: 41.6 g; Dietary Fiber: 3.6 g; Sugars: 4.1 g; Protein: 5.3 g; Cholesterol: 0 mg; Sodium: 501.3 mg

70. __Almond Flour Pancakes__

Yield: 3 Servings
Total Time: 30 Minutes
Prep Time:10 Minutes
Cook Time: 20 Minutes

Ingredients:
- Almond Flour (1¾ cups)
- Baking Powder (1 tsp.)
- Tapioca Flour (2 tbsp.)
- Salt (1/4 tsp.)
- Eggs (2, lightly beaten)
- Vanilla Extract (1 tsp.)
- Almond Milk (3/4 cup)

Directions
Add all your wet ingredients to a medium bowl and whisk to combine. Add your dry ingredients and gently mix until fully combined and smooth.

Tip: Consider setting batter in the refrigerator for a few minutes before cooking to allow the batter to become thicker in texture.

Set your electric pressure cooker on 'sauté' mode, lightly greased with oil, and allow to heat up. Pour in your batter. Close the lid, and switch the cooking modes to 'manual' and set to cook on low pressure for 45 minutes.

When the timer goes off perform a quick release, by pressing 'cancel' then carefully turning the pressure valve to venting. **Tip:** Consider using a pot holder, or long spoon to turn the valve as it will be extremely hot. Carefully open, and ease out with a spatula. Slice, serve and enjoy your favorite pancake syrup.

Nutritional Information per Serving:
Calories: 270; Total Fat: 15 g; Carbs: 32 g; Dietary Fiber: 1 g;
Sugars: 14 g; Protein: 3 g; Cholesterol: 0 mg; Sodium: 340 mg

71. Almond Flour Naan Bread & Spicy Avocado

Yield: 2 Servings
Total Time: 40 Minutes
Prep Time:10 Minutes
Cook Time: 30 Minutes

Ingredients
- Almond Flour (1/2 cup)
- Tapioca Flour (1/2 cup)
- Coconut Milk (1 cup)
- Salt (1 tsp.)
- Avocado (2)
- Red Chili Pepper (1 tbsp., flakes)

Directions:
Combine all your ingredients in a large bowl. Set your 9.5-inch non-stick pan over medium heat.

Tip: Consider setting batter in the refrigerator for a few minutes before cooking to allow the batter to become thicker in texture.

Set your electric pressure cooker on 'sauté' mode, lightly greased with oil, and allow to heat up. Pour in your batter. Close the lid, and switch the cooking modes to 'manual' and set to cook on low pressure for 45 minutes.
When the timer goes off perform a quick release, by pressing 'cancel' then carefully turning the pressure valve to venting.
Tip: Consider using a pot holder, or long spoon to turn the valve as it will be extremely hot.
Meanwhile, dice and peel avocado. Transfer avocado to a small bowl, combine spices in a bowl and stir in your avocado. Carefully open, serve naan with avocado.

Nutritional Information per Serving:
Calories: 142; Total Fat: 15.8 g; Carbs: 17.5 g; Dietary Fiber: 12.1 g; Sugars: 1.4 g; Protein: 3.3g; Cholesterol:71 mg; Sodium: 160 mg

72. Coconut Flour Waffles

Yield: 2 Servings
Total Time: 30 Minutes
Prep Time:10 Minutes
Cook Time: 20 Minutes

Ingredients:
- Coconut Flour (1 cups)
- Salt (1/4 tsp.)
- Baking Soda (1/4 tsp.)
- Eggs (4)
- Vanilla (1 tsp.)
- Stevia (2 tbsp.)
- Cinnamon (1/4 tsp.)

Directions
Add all your wet ingredients to a medium bowl and whisk to combine. Add your dry ingredients and gently mix until fully combined and smooth.

Tip: Consider setting batter in the refrigerator for a few minutes before cooking to allow the batter to become thicker in texture.

Set your electric pressure cooker on 'sauté' mode, lightly greased with oil, and allow to heat up. Pour in your batter. Close the lid, and switch the cooking modes to 'manual' and set to cook on low pressure for 45 minutes.

When the timer goes off perform a quick release, by pressing 'cancel' then carefully turning the pressure valve to venting. **Tip:** Consider using a pot holder, or long spoon to turn the valve as it will be extremely hot. Carefully open, and ease out with a spatula.
Slice, serve, and enjoy with maple syrup.

Nutritional Information per Serving:

Calories: 89; Total Fat: 6.2 g; Carbs: 16.1 g; Dietary Fiber: 0.6 g; Sugars: 0.6 g; Protein: 5 g; Cholesterol: 309 mg; Sodium: 1215 mg

73. <u>Blueberry Corn Muffins</u>

Yield: 6 Servings
Total Time: 40 Minutes
Prep Time: 20 Minutes
Cook Time: 20 Minutes

Ingredients

- Almond Flour (1/2 cups)
- Coconut Flour (1/4 cup)
- Salt (1/4 tsp.)
- Baking Soda (1/4 tsp.)
- Eggs (3, large)
- Oil (1/4 cup)
- Stevia (3 tbsp.)
- Coconut Milk (1/4 cup)
- Blueberries (3/4 cup, fresh)

Directions

Add all your dry ingredients of the muffin to your electric mixer bowl. In a separate bowl, combine all your muffin's wet ingredients in a separate bowl, then to your dry ingredients and allow to whisk on low until fully combined. Fold in your blueberries, and set aside. Fit your Electric pressure cooker with your steel insert, and a trivet then add your water and set the cooker on the sauté setting to allow it to preheat.

Fill up silicone muffin cups ⅔ way full with your muffin batter and set your muffin cups to set on top of the trivet you fitted into the cooker. Prep a cover by cutting a piece of parchment paper and aluminum foil to create a circle then use to cover your muffin cups.

Set your Electric pressure cooker to pressure on high for 8 minutes. Once your timer has finished, press 'cancel' and allow your cooker to cook down naturally for about 15 to 20 minutes before attempting to open. Test your muffins for doneness as you would a cake. Cool, serve, and enjoy!

Nutritional Information per Serving:
Calories: 234; Total Fat: 20.2 g; Carbs: 18.2 g; Dietary Fiber: 2.4 g;
Sugars: 8 g; Protein: 4.5 g; Cholesterol: 92 mg; Sodium: 114 mg

74. <u>Almond Flour Cornbread</u>

Yield: 9 Servings
Total Time 20 Minutes
Prep Time:10 Minutes
Cook Time: 10 Minutes

Ingredients
- Almond Flour (1/2 cup)
- Coconut Flour (1/4 cup)
- Salt (1/4 tsp.)
- Baking Soda (1/4 tsp.)
- Eggs (3)
- Butter (1/4 cup, unsalted, melted)
- Honey (2 tbsp.)
- Almond Milk (1/2 cup)

Directions
Add your almond milk, honey, butter, and eggs. Whisk to combine then set aside. In a separate bowl, add your baking soda, salt, coconut flour, and almond flour, then stir.
Pour your batter into your prepared pan (preferably 7-inches or smaller).

Fit your Electric pressure cooker with your steel insert, and a trivet then add your water and set the cooker on the sauté setting to allow it to preheat. Prep a cover by cutting a piece of parchment paper and aluminum foil to create a circle then use to cover your muffin cups.

Set your Electric pressure cooker to pressure on high for 8 minutes. Once your timer has finished, press 'cancel' and allow your cooker to cook down naturally for about 15 to 20 minutes before attempting to open. Carefully open, cool slightly, and serve.

Nutritional Information per Serving:
Calories: 58; Total Fat: 5 g; Carbs: 3 g; Dietary Fiber: 0 g;
Sugars: 1.4 g; Protein: 2 g; Cholesterol: 2 mg; Sodium: 134 mg

75. **Pumpkin Spice Bread**

Yields: 2 loaves
Total Time 20 Minutes
Prep Time:10 Minutes
Cook Time: 10 Minutes

Ingredients
- Almond Flour (1 cup)
- Sea Salt (1/4 tsp.)
- Baking Soda (1/2 tsp.)
- Cinnamon (2 tbsp., ground)
- Nutmeg (2 tsp., ground)
- Cloves (1 tsp., ground)
- Ginger (1 tsp., ground)
- Allspice (1 tsp. ground)
- Eggs (3)
- Butter (1/4 cup, unsalted, melted)
- Honey (2 tbsp.)
- Almond Milk (1/2 cup)
- Pumpkin Puree (1/4 cup)

Directions
In a large bowl, combine your allspice, ginger, cloves, nutmeg, cinnamon, baking soda, salt, and almond flour. Add your pumpkin, milk, honey, butter, eggs in a medium bowl. Whisk to combine, and add wet ingredients to dry bowl. Pour your batter into your prepared pan (preferably 7-inches or smaller).

Fit your Electric pressure cooker with your steel insert, and a trivet then add your water and set the cooker on the sauté setting to allow it to preheat. Prep a cover by cutting a piece of parchment paper and aluminum foil to create a circle then use to cover your muffin cups.

Set your Electric pressure cooker to pressure on high for 8 minutes. Once your timer has finished, press 'cancel' and allow your cooker to cook down naturally for about 15 to 20 minutes before attempting to open. Carefully open, cool, slice and serve.

Nutritional Information per Serving:
Calories: 365; Total Fat: 30 g; Carbs: 19.2 g; Dietary Fiber: 6 g; Sugars: 4 g; Protein: 13 g; Cholesterol: 344 mg; Sodium: 537 mg

76. <u>Gluten Free Nutty Bread</u>

Yields: 2 loaves
Total Time 20 Minutes
Prep Time:10 Minutes
Cook Time: 10 Minutes

Ingredients
- Eggs (2)
- Sour cream (1/4 cup)
- Honey (1/4 cup)
- Lemon Juice (1 tsp.)
- Almond Flour (3 cups)
- Baking Soda (1 tsp.)
- Sea Salt (1/8 tsp.)
- Walnuts (1/2 cup, chopped)

Directions
In a large bowl, add walnuts, salt, baking soda, almond flour, then stir to combine. Combine all your wet ingredients in a separate bowl, and whisk until fully combined. Add your remaining dry ingredients and whisk to combine. Pour your batter into your prepared pan (preferably 7-inches or smaller).

Fit your Electric pressure cooker with your steel insert, and a trivet then add your water and set the cooker on the sauté setting to allow it to preheat. Prep a cover by cutting a piece of parchment paper and aluminum foil to create a circle then use to cover your muffin cups.

Set your Electric pressure cooker to pressure on high for 8 minutes. Once your timer has finished, press 'cancel' and allow your cooker to cook down naturally for about 15 to 20 minutes before attempting to open. Carefully open, cool, slice and serve.

Nutritional Information per Serving:
Calories: 304; Total Fat: 27.3 g; Carbs: 23.4 g; Dietary Fiber: 2.1 g; Sugars: 2 g; Protein: 10.2 g; Cholesterol: 319 mg; Sodium: 231 mg

77. **<u>Almond Flour Tortilla</u>**

Yields:6 serving
Total Time: 25 Minutes
Prep Time:10 Minutes
Cook Time: 15 Minutes

Ingredients:
- Almond Flour (2 cups)
- Eggs (2)
- Olive Oil (1 tsp.)
- Sea Salt (1/2 tsp.)

Directions:
Add all your ingredients to a medium bowl and stir with a wooden spoon or knead with hands to combine.

Tip: Consider setting batter in the refrigerator for a few minutes before cooking to allow the batter to become thicker in texture.

Divide into 6 even portions, and roll out to desired thickness. Lay in a single layer on your electric pressure cooker, and layer with trivets. Close the lid, and set to cook on 'manual' for 6 minutes.

Allow your cooker to cook down naturally for about 15 to 20 minutes before attempting to open. Carefully open, and serve as is for a side or top with desired toppings for tacos. Enjoy!

Nutritional Information per Serving:
Calories: 29; Total Fat: 2.5 g; Carbs: 0 g; Dietary Fiber: 0 g; Sugars: 0 g; Protein: 1.5 g; Cholesterol: 103 mg; Sodium: 211 mg

78. <u>Almond Crusted Baked</u> <u>Zucchini Crisps</u>

Yields: 4 serving
Total Time: 15 Minutes
Prep Time:10 Minutes
Cook Time: 5 Minutes

Ingredients:
- Zucchini (1 large, sliced)
- Almond Flour (1 cup)
- Egg (1 large)
- Salt (1 tsp.)
- Garlic Powder (1 tsp.)
- Thyme (1 tsp.)
- Black Pepper (1/4 tsp.)

Directions
Crack your egg in a small bowl and lightly beat. Combine your flour, seasoning, and spices in a separate bowl. Dip your zucchini piece in your egg, drain excess and then transfer to your flour mixture to coat.

Set your electric pressure cooker with oil to preheat on 'sauté' mode. Place the zucchini in a single layer on your electric pressure cooker, and brown on both sides. Close your lid, and set to cook on 'manual' for 1 minute.

When the timer goes off perform a quick release, by pressing 'cancel' then carefully turning the pressure valve to venting. **Tip:** Consider using a pot holder, or long spoon to turn the valve as it will be extremely hot. Carefully open, serve, and enjoy!

Nutritional Information per Serving:
Calories: 230; Total Fat: 19.1 g; Carbs: 10 g; Dietary Fiber: 5 g; Sugars: 1 g; Protein: 9 g; Cholesterol: 46 mg; Sodium: 587 mg

79. Almond Sweet and Sour Cauliflower

Yields: 6 serving
Total Time: 15 Minutes
Prep Time:10 Minutes
Cook Time: 5 Minutes

Ingredients
- 3 lbs. cauliflower (cut into bite size)
- 2 tsp. salt
- 3 cloves garlic (chopped)
- 1 tbsp. chopped onion
- 1 tsp. black pepper
- 4 oz. almond flour
- 1 L. oil (for frying)
- 1 ½ cup water
- ½ cup vinegar
- ¾ lb. sugar
- 5 slices ginger
- ½ cup tomato ketchup
- 2 tbsp. cornstarch

Directions:
Wash and drain cauliflower. Season with garlic, onion, salt, and pepper. Use almond flour to coat cauliflower pieces and deep fry. Set cooked cauliflower aside.

Combine water, ketchup, vinegar, and sugar in an electric pressure cooker on 'sauté' mode. Add ginger slices and stir to combine. Mix out cornstarch in a small amount of water and stir in the mixture to thicken the sauce. Close lid and set to cook on 'manual' mode for 5 minutes.

When the timer goes off perform a quick release, by pressing 'cancel' then carefully turning the pressure valve to venting. **Tip:** Consider using a pot holder, or long spoon to turn the valve as it will be extremely hot. Pour sauce over cauliflower, and stir to coat evenly. Serve and enjoy.

Nutritional Information per Serving:
Calories: 262; Total Fat: 10.1 g; Carbs: 21 g; Dietary Fiber: 7.3 g; Sugars: 24.2 g; Protein: 9 g; Cholesterol: 0 mg; Sodium: 847 mg

80. Almond Mustard Glazed Brussel Sprouts

Yields: 6 serving
Total Time: 1 Hour 10 Minutes
Prep Time: 10 Minutes
Cook Time: 1 Hour

Ingredients

- 3 lbs. brussel sprouts
- 4 oz. almond flour
- 1 tsp. salt
- ½ tsp. paprika
- 1 tsp. white pepper
- ½ tsp. garlic powder
- ½ cup soft margarine
- ½ cup mustard
- 6 tsp. lime juice
- ½ tsp. salt

Directions

Wash and drain brussel sprouts. Use a clean cloth or paper towel to dry. In a paper bag, combine salt, almond flour, paprika, chicken seasoning and white pepper. Put brussel sprouts in the bag and shake vigorously to coat properly.

Set your electric pressure cooker on 'sauté' mode with margarine, and allow to heat up. Once melted, roll brussel sprouts in melted margarine until all sides are coated. Fix the brussel sprouts in the electric pressure cooker, packing them close to each other but not overcrowded. Stir brussel sprouts and pour on glaze.

Close the lid, and set to cook on 'manual' mode with low pressure for 30 minutes. When the timer goes off perform a quick release, by pressing 'cancel' then carefully turning the pressure valve to venting. **Tip:** Consider using a pot holder, or long spoon to turn the valve as it will be extremely hot. Carefully open, mix all ingredients together and serve.

Nutritional Information per Serving:
Calories: 360; Total Fat: 26 g; Carbs: 26.8 g; Dietary Fiber: 12 g; Sugars: 7 g; Protein: 13 g; Cholesterol: 0 mg; Sodium: 1001 mg

81. Almond Dusted Baked Tofu

Yields: 4 serving
Total Time: 55 Minutes
Prep Time: 10 Minutes
Cook Time: 45 Minutes

Ingredients

- 2 lbs. tofu, extra firm
- 1 tbsp. lemon/lime juice
- 1 egg (beaten)
- 6 tsp. milk
- 6 tsp. butter
- 6 tsp. almond flour
- 3 pimento seeds (crushed)
- ½ tsp. salt
- ½ tsp. black pepper
- 6 okra (sliced)
- 1 tomato (sliced)

Directions

Drain your tofu, and wrap in a clean towel. Lay your wrapped tofu on a flat surface, and top with a heavy pan for about 10 minutes. Unwrap, and cut your tofu into cubes. Sprinkle with lemon/lime juice and season with salt, crushed pimento, and pepper

Place in a greased, baking dish.

Pour milk into your electric pressure cooker. Brush the tofu with egg, sprinkle almond flour over it. Put dots of butter. Arrange okra and tomato slices atop tofu. Close the lid, and allow to cook on 'pressure' mode for 10 minutes with low pressure.

When the timer goes off perform a quick release, by pressing 'cancel' then carefully turning the pressure valve to venting.

Tip: Consider using a pot holder, or long spoon to turn the valve as it will be extremely hot. Carefully open, mix all ingredients together and serve.

Nutritional Information per Serving: Calories: 456; Total Fat: 34.1 g; Carbs: 22.8 g; Dietary Fiber: 8.4 g; Sugars: 7 g; Protein: 21 g; Cholesterol: 56 mg; Sodium: 100.1 mg

82. <u>CHAPTER 8: Dessert Recipes</u>

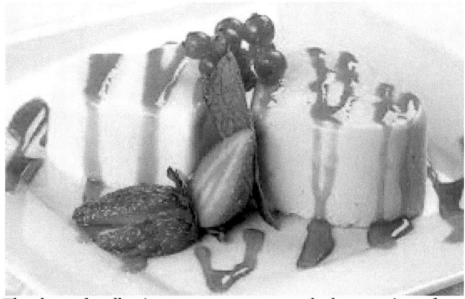

Thank you for allowing us to expose you to the large variety of Keto Vegetarian recipes that you can enjoy, please feel free to leave us a positive review if you like what you are about to read through.

83. <u>Strawberry Almond Bundt Cake</u>

Yields: 12 serving
Total Time: 1hr 40min
Prep Time: 10 Minutes
Cook Time: 1hr 30min

Ingredients:
- 1 lb. coconut sugar
- 6 tbsp. butter

- 1 lb. almond flour
- 4 tsp. baking powder
- 1 tsp. salt
- 1 pt. strawberry
- 1 pt. evaporated milk

Directions

Grease and line a 10 in. Bundt pan. Preheat oven to 325 degrees F. Combine almond flour, baking powder, and salt. Lay aside. Cream 1 lb. of sugar and 6 tbsp. butter until really fluffy in a large container. Fold in flour mixture, alternate with evaporated milk.
Mix in cranberries and pour mixture into greased pan.

Bake in prepared oven for an hour. When cake is baked, a toothpick inserted should come out clean. Allow 10 mins. for cooling then turn out on a wire rack, let it remain until totally cooled. Serve and enjoy.

Nutritional Information per Serving:
Calories: 310; Total Fat: 26 g; Carbs: 13.4 g; Dietary Fiber: 5.6 g; Sugars: 6 g; Protein: 10 g; Cholesterol: 19 mg; Sodium: 297 mg

84. **Moist Almond Cake**

Yields: 8 serving
Total Time: 1hr 10min
Prep Time: 10 Minutes
Cook Time: 1 Hour

Ingredients
- 2 oz. butter (soft)
- 5 oz. sugar
- 1 cup almond flour
- 1 tsp. baking powder
- ¼ tsp. baking soda
- ¼ tsp. salt
- ½ tsp. cinnamon powder
- 1 tsp. vanilla
- 1 egg
- 1 cup Greek yogurt, vanilla (full fat)

Directions
Grease a 9-inch layer cake tin and sprinkle with a little almond flour. Heat oven to 375 degrees F. Sift your cinnamon powder, salt, baking soda, baking powder, almond flour, and sugar in a large bowl. Stir to combine, and set aside.

Place in a blender, egg, butter, sugar, banana, and vanilla. Blend for 1 minute at super speed; consistency should be smooth. Pour blended mixture into almond flour mixture and mix thoroughly.

Pour and scrape into greased tin. Place in oven and bake for 25 mins. Cool and serve.

Nutritional Information per Serving:
Calories: 157; Total Fat: 8 g; Carbs: 19.5 g; Dietary Fiber: 0.1 g; Sugars: 19 g; Protein: 2.3 g; Cholesterol: 97 mg; Sodium: 187 mg

85. <u>Coconut Cobbler</u>

Yield: 6 Servings
Total Time: 55 Minutes
Prep Time:10 Minutes
Cook Time: 45 Minutes

Ingredients:

Coconut Layer
- Coconut (1 cup, toasted, shredded)
- Cinnamon (1/2 tsp.)
- Coconut Sugar (1 tbsp.)
- Coconut Flakes (1 tbsp.)
- Arrowroot Powder (1/2 tsp.)

Cobbler Layer
- Almond Milk (1/2 cup)
- Coconut Oil (1/4 cup, melted)
- Vanilla Extract (1/2 tsp)
- Almond Flour (1/2 cup)
- Arrowroot Powder (1/3 cup)
- Baking Powder (1 tsp.)
- Cinnamon (1 tsp.)
- Sea Salt (1 tsp.)

Topping
- Coconut Flakes (1 tbsp., unsweetened)
- Cinnamon (1 tbsp.)

Directions

Set your oven to preheat to 375 degrees F, and prepare a skillet by lightly greasing it with coconut oil. Add all your coconut layer ingredients to a medium bowl and lightly stir to fully combine, then add to your prepared skillet.

Next, combine all your crumble layer ingredients in another medium bowl, then spoon onto the coconut layer. Set to bake until done (about 25 minutes, test just you would a cake with a toothpick). Top with coconut flakes, and cinnamon, then serve.

Nutritional Information per Serving:
Calories: 103; Total Fat: 8.3 g; Carbs: 7.1 g; Dietary Fiber: 1.2 g; Sugars: 4.9 g; Protein: 1.1 g; Cholesterol: 39 mg; Sodium: 62 mg

86. Almond Butter Cup Cookies

Yield: 12 Cookies
Total Time: 1 Hour 40 Minutes
Prep Time:10 Minutes
Cook Time: 90 Minutes

Ingredients:
- Almond Butter (1 cup)
- Coconut Crystals (1/2 cup)
- Vanilla Extract (1 tsp.)
- Almond Extract (1/4 tsp.)
- Eggs (2)
- Almond Flour (1/2 cup, blanched)
- Coconut Flour (2 tbsp.)
- Salt (1/4 tsp.)
- Dark Chocolate (1 cup, chopped, unsweetened)

Directions
Set your oven to preheat to 350 degrees F, and prepare a baking sheet by lightly greasing it with coconut oil. Combine your coconut crystals, almond butter, eggs, almond extract, and vanilla extract in a medium bowl.

Next, combine your flours, and salt in another bowl, then add them to your wet ingredients and fold until fully combined. Begin to form your cookies by taking a golf ball sized ball of dough and forming into peanut butter cups.

Place your cookies on your baking sheet and allow to bake for about 12 minutes (cookies should easily lift off the baking sheet when done). Chill for about 30 minutes in the refrigerator. While your cookies are chilling, melt your chocolate over medium heat, in a double boiler, then cool for at least 15 minutes.

Pour on top of your chilled cookies, then allow to freeze until your chocolate rehardens (about 30 minutes). Serve, and enjoy.

Nutritional Information per Serving:
Calories: 137.4; Total Fat: 11.8 g; Carbs: 8.6 g; Dietary Fiber: 2.3 g;
Sugars: 1.3 g; Protein: 4.1 g; Cholesterol: 0.6 mg; Sodium: 56.8 mg

87. <u>Pumpkin Almond Cake</u>

Yields: 12 serving
Total Time: 1hr 40min
Prep Time: 10 Minutes
Cook Time: 1hr 30min

Ingredients:
- 1 lb. coconut sugar
- 6 tbsp. butter
- 1 lb. almond flour
- 4 tsp. baking powder
- 1 tsp. salt
- 1 cup pumpkin puree
- 1 tsp. Cinnamon
- ¼ tsp. nutmeg
- 1 pt. evaporated milk

Directions

Grease and line a 10 in. Bundt pan. Preheat oven to 325 degrees F. Combine almond flour, baking powder, and salt. Lay aside. Cream 1 lb. of sugar and 6 tbsp. butter until really fluffy in a large container. Fold in flour mixture, alternate with evaporated milk.
Mix in cranberries and pour mixture into greased pan.

Bake in prepared oven for an hour. When cake is baked, a toothpick inserted should come out clean. Allow 10 mins. for cooling then turn out on a wire rack, let it remain until totally cooled. Serve and enjoy.

Nutritional Information per Serving:
Calories: 359; Total Fat: 31 g; Carbs: 13.1 g; Dietary Fiber: 6 g; Sugars: 5 g; Protein: 12.5 g; Cholesterol: 19 mg; Sodium: 322 mg

88. __Gluten Free Dark Chocolate Cake__

Yield: 12 Servings
Total Time: 1 Hour 5 Minutes
Prep Time:10 Minutes
Cook Time: 55 Minutes

Ingredients:
- Almond flour (2 cups)
- Tapioca Flour (1 tbsp.)
- Stevia (1 cup)
- Unsweetened cocoa (¾ cup)
- Baking soda (2 tsp.)
- Baking powder (1 tsp.)
- Salt (½ tsp.)
- Eggs (2)
- Chocolate yogurt (1 cup, full fat)
- Milk (1 cup)
- Vegetable oil (½ cup)
- Vinegar (2 tsp.)

Directions:
Grease and flour a 9x13-inch pan. Preheat oven to 350 degrees F. Combine the first six ingredients in a large bowl. Make a well in the center and pour the last five ingredients from the list and mix until smooth.

Put the batter into the 9x13 inch pan. Bake for 40 minutes in the oven, or until a toothpick comes out clean after sticking into the center of the cake. Allow the cake to cool. Serve and enjoy!

Nutritional Information per Serving:
Calories: 340; Total Fat: 13 g; Carbs: 52 g; Dietary Fiber: 2 g; Sugars: 40 g; Protein: 3 g; Cholesterol: 30 mg; Sodium: 310 mg

89. __Vanilla Almond Cake__

Yields: 12 serving
Total Time: 55 Minutes
Prep Time:10 Minutes
Cook Time: 45 Minutes

Ingredients
- Milk (2 cups)
- Egg yolks (6)
- Almond Flour (7 ½ tablespoons)
- Frozen puff pastry (17.5 oz)
- Vanilla bean (1 whole)
- Apricot preserves (1/2 cup)
- Castor sugar (3/4 cup)
- Almond (1 cup, sliced)
- Salt

Directions
Bring milk to a boil in a saucepan then put in vanilla bean. Remove from heat and allow to cool until warm. Combine sugar, yolks, flour, and salt in another saucepan then slowly add warm milk and whisk to combine. Cook over a medium-low flame until mixture thickens, stirring constantly with a wooden spoon. Put custard in a bowl and cool, stirring occasionally.

Set oven to 400°F. Lay pastry sheet in a 14*17 baking sheet about a half inch thick. Use a fork to poke dough all over. Bake for 28 minutes then take from oven and cool.
Take cooled pastry from baking sheet and cut into 3 (5" wide strips). Use custard to top strip then add another strip on top and top with jam then top with a third strip and sprinkle with almond slices. Cut into 8 pieces and serve.

Nutritional Information per Serving:
Calories: 324; Total Fat: 22 g; Carbs: 34 g; Dietary Fiber: 2.1 g; Sugars: 5.7 g; Protein: 7.2 g; Cholesterol: 55 mg; Sodium: 131 mg

90. Gluten Free Cheesecake Chocolate Squares

Yield: 16 Servings
Total Time: 1 Hour 5 Minutes
Prep Time:10 Minutes
Cook Time: 55 Minutes

Ingredients:
- Cream cheese (1 package, softened)
- Coconut sugar (3/4 cup)
- Egg (1)
- Semisweet chocolate chips (2 cups)
- Butter (¼ cup)
- Eggs (2)
- Almond flour (2/3 cup)
- Baking powder (½ tsp.)
- Salt (¼ tsp.)

Directions:
Grease a 9-inch square baking pan. Preheat oven to 350 degrees F. Combine the first three ingredients, and a cup of chocolate chips in a large mixing bowl, and whisk until smooth. Set aside.

Set your remaining chocolate chips, and butter to melt in a double boiler.
Add your remaining ingredients to your melted chocolate mixture and stir until fully combined. In the baking pan pour both batters in layers starting with the chocolate.

Bake for 30 minutes in the oven or until edges pull away from both side of the pan and top is crinkled. Let it cool completely. Slice into squares, serve and enjoy!

Nutritional Information per Serving:
Calories: 222; Total Fat: 20 g; Carbs: 6 g; Dietary Fiber: 1 g;
Sugars: 2 g; Protein: 4 g; Cholesterol:71 mg; Sodium: 160 mg

91. **Sugar Free Maple Donuts**

Yield: 6 Servings
Total Time: 1 Hour
Prep Time:10 Minutes
Cook Time: 50 Minutes

Ingredients
- Almond Flour (1 ¾ cups)
- Coconut Flour (2 tbsp.)
- Baking Soda (1 tsp.)
- Cinnamon (2 tsp.)
- Eggs (4)
- Maple Syrup (1/3 cups, sugar free)
- Coconut Oil (1/4 cup, melted)
- Vanilla Extract (2 tsp.)
- Coconut Butter (1/4 cup)
- Coconut Milk (1/4 cup, full-fat, shaken)
- Butter (2 tbsp., grass-fed)
- Dijon Mustard (1 tbsp.)

Directions:
Set your oven to preheat to 350 degrees F, and prepare a donut pan by lightly greasing with coconut oil. Sift together your flours, 1 tsp. cinnamon, and baking soda in a large bowl. To your flour mixture, add your eggs, 1 tsp. vanilla, coconut oil, and ½ cup maple
syrup. Mix until the mixture becomes smooth.

Spoon your donut batter into a large piping bag, and cut the tip ¾ inches from the point. Pipe your batter into your donut cavity then set to bake until done (about 20 minutes). Prepare a glaze by adding coconut butter, maple syrup, 1 tsp. cinnamon, 1 tsp. vanilla, butter, and coconut butter in a blender then pulsing until smooth. Transfer your glaze to a shallow bowl then set aside.

Once your donuts are done adjust your oven to 375 degrees F, then prepare a baking sheet by lining it with aluminum foil. Drizzle with donut glaze, serve, and enjoy!

Nutritional Information per Serving:

Calories: 270; Total Fat: 15 g; Carbs: 32 g; Dietary Fiber: 1 g; Sugars: 14 g; Protein: 3 g; Cholesterol: 0 mg; Sodium: 340 mg

92. <u>**Almond Rock Buns**</u>

Yields: 6 serving
Total Time: 55 Minutes
Prep Time: 10 Minutes
Cook Time: 45 Minutes

Ingredients
- 4 oz. almond flour
- 2 tsp. baking powder
- ½ cup brown sugar
- 3 oz. margarine (hard)
- ½ tsp. grated nutmeg
- ½ tsp. mixed spice
- 1 tsp. vanilla
- 4 tbsp. grated coconut
- 1 egg
- 2 tbsp. milk

Directions
Sift together flour, salt, baking powder and spices in a bowl. Cut in margarine and crumble with fingertips or pastry blender. Add fruits, grated coconut, beaten egg, and milk. Mix together to make a stiff dough. Pile in rough heaps on a greased baking tray.
Bake at 350 degrees F for about 20 mins. Serve, and enjoy.

Nutritional Information per Serving:
Calories: 131; Total Fat: 5.7 g; Carbs: 18.7 g; Dietary Fiber: 0.6 g; Sugars: 3.5 g; Protein: 2.2 g; Cholesterol: 13.6 mg; Sodium: 93.3 mg

93. <u>Lemon Chocolate Chip Squares</u>

Yield: 24 Servings
Total Time: 50 Minutes
Prep Time:10 Minutes
Cook Time: 40 Minutes

Ingredients:
- Butter (3/4 cup)
- Coconut sugar (1 cup)
- Egg (1, beaten)
- Vanilla extract (1tsp.)
- Lemon Zest (1 tbsp.)
- Almond flour (1 3/4 cups)
- Baking powder (2 tsp.)
- Salt (1/2 tsp.)
- Semisweet chocolate chips (1 cup)

Directions:
Grease and flour a 10x15 inch jelly roll pan. Preheat oven to 350 degrees F. Cream together your butter and sugar, in a large bowl, until fluffy. Add your egg and vanilla and continue whisking until combined.

Next and in your bananas and fold. Once combined, add in your remaining ingredients and fold until the mixture forms a smooth batter. Spoon the mixture into your jelly roll pan, and bake until set (about 20 minutes). Cool, and cut into 24 even squares. Serve, and enjoy!

Nutritional Information per Serving:
Calories: 156.4; Total Fat: 7.5 g; Carbs: 21.4g; Dietary Fiber: 0.8 g; Sugars: 14.6 g; Protein: 1.9 g; Cholesterol: 40 mg; Sodium: 81.6 mg

94. **Coconut Bread Pudding**

Yields: 4 serving
Total Time: 1 Hour 30 Minutes
Prep Time: 10 Minutes
Cook Time: 1 Hour 20 Minutes

Ingredients
For Coconut Sauce
- Butter (1/4 lb.)
- Sugar (1/2 cup)
- Coconut Water (4 tablespoons)

For Bread Pudding
- French Bread (6oz)
- Butter (1 tablespoon)
- Egg (1)
- Sugar (3/4 cup sugar)
- Silvered almonds (2 tablespoons)
- Vanilla Extract (1/8 teaspoon)
- Raisins (2 tablespoons)
- Milk Powder (2 tablespoons)
- Coconut Water (2 cups)

Directions
Set oven to 300F/150C. In a pan, mix sugar, egg, vanilla extract, coconut water, and milk powder. Set the bread pieces in a baking pan and cover with raisins, pour the mixture to cover the bread and place in oven for 50mins.

Prepare the coconut sauce by combining sugar, butter and coconut water in a saucepan, and heat until the mixture is blended correctly. Remove the bread pudding from the oven and pour the coconut sauce on top and serve while warm.

Nutritional Information per Serving:
Calories: 291; Total Fat: 8.8 g; Carbs: 45.03 g; Dietary Fiber: 1.8 g; Sugars: 41.11 g; Protein: 7.55 g; Cholesterol: 15 mg; Sodium: 451 mg

95. Dairy-Free Vegan Pumpkin Almond Cupcakes

Yields: 12 serving
Total Time: 45 Minutes
Prep Time: 10 Minutes
Cook Time: 35 Minutes

Ingredients

- Almond milk (1/4 cup)
- Cider vinegar (1 teaspoon)
- Almond flour (1 ¼ cup)
- Baking powder (1 teaspoon)
- Baking soda (1/2 teaspoon)
- Stevia (1/2 cup)
- Cashews (1/4 cup, ground finely)
- Cinnamon (1 teaspoon)
- Ginger (1/2 teaspoon)
- Nutmeg (1/2 teaspoon)
- Salt (1/2 teaspoon)
- Pumpkin (1/2 cup, pureed)
- Canola oil (1/3 cup)
- Sour cream (2 teaspoons, dairy free)
- Vanilla extract (1 teaspoon)

Directions

Preheat oven to 350° F. In a small bowl, mix vinegar and almond milk together and set aside for 5 minutes. Mix baking powder, flour, baking soda, cinnamon, cashews, nutmeg, ginger, and salt together in a large bowl. Using another bowl mix canola oil, pumpkin puree, vanilla, sour cream and vinegar mixture together. Add liquid mixture to dry ingredients and combine. Line muffin tin with paper liners and t batter into molds about 2/3 full. Allow to bake for 20 minutes, then remove from heat and allow to cool then top with desired frosting.

Nutritional Information per Serving: Calories: 202; Total Fat: 10.3 g; Carbs: 36.9 g; Dietary Fiber: 2 g; Sugars: 10.6 g; Protein: 2 g; Cholesterol: 0 mg; Sodium: 205.7 mg

96. **Almond Flour Pudding**

Yield: 6 Servings
Total Time: 1 Hour
Prep Time:10 Minutes
Cook Time: 40 Minutes

Ingredients:
- Butter (½ cup, melted)
- Stevia (1/2 cup)
- Almond flour (1 cup)
- Baking powder (2 tsp.)
- Salt (¼ tsp.)
- Milk (1 cup)
- Ground cinnamon (1 tsp.)

Directions:
Set your oven to preheat to 375 degrees F, and lightly grease an 8-inch cake tin. Put the first seven ingredients in a bowl and whisk until smooth.

Pour your batter into your prepared cake tin and set to bake until golden (about 30 minutes). Serve and enjoy!

Nutritional Information per Serving:
Calories: 127.9; Total Fat: 4.2 g; Carbs: 22.3 g; Dietary Fiber: 2.1 g; Sugars: 13.5 g; Protein: 3.4 g; Cholesterol: 34.9 mg; Sodium: 147.2 mg

97. <u>Red Velvet Cupcakes</u>

Yields: 12 serving
Total Time: 40 Minutes
Prep Time: 10 Minutes
Cook Time: 30 Minutes

Ingredients
- Almond Milk (1 cup)
- Baking soda (1/2 teaspoon)
- Apple Cider Vinegar (1 teaspoon)
- Coconut Flour (1 ¼ cups)
- Coconut Sugar (1 cup)
- Cocoa powder (2 tablespoons)
- Baking powder (1/2 teaspoon)
- Salt (½ teaspoon)
- Canola Oil (1/3 cup)
- Red Food Coloring (2 tablespoons)
- Vanilla Extract (2 teaspoons)
- Almond Extract (1/4 teaspoon)

Directions
Preheat the oven to 350°F. Combine vinegar and milk and put to the side to allow the mix to curdle. Sift cocoa powder, flour, baking soda, salt and baking powder in a large bowl. Add oil, extracts and food coloring to curdled milk and whisk. Make a hole in the center of the dry ingredients and add liquid mixture to it. Stir to combine. Try not to over mix. Line muffin tin with paper liners and fill each mold about 2/3 full for each. Bake for 20 minutes and remove from heat. Cool and add the desired frosting.

Nutritional Information per Serving:
Calories: 290.1; Total Fat: 10.6 g; Carbs: 47.9 g; Dietary Fiber: 1 g; Sugars: 36.2 g; Protein: 2.5 g; Cholesterol: 0 mg; Sodium: 199.8 mg

98. Vegan Blueberry Cupcakes

Yields: 12 serving
Total Time: 40 Minutes
Prep Time: 10 Minutes
Cook Time: 30 Minutes

Ingredients
- Dairy free soy margarine (3/4 cups, softened)
- Coconut sugar (1 ½ cup)
- Soy yogurt-vanilla (1/4 cup)
- Vanilla (2 teaspoons)
- Silken tofu (1/4 cup, pureed)
- Coconut flour (2 cups)
- Baking powder (1 teaspoon)
- Salt (1 teaspoon)
- Coconut milk (1 cup)
- Blueberries-fresh (1 cup, crushed)

Directions
Preheat the oven to 350° F. Using a mixer, cream butter, and sugar for about 4 minutes until fluffy. Then add tofu, vanilla, and yogurt and blend until the mix becomes creamy. Set mixture aside. Sift baking powder, flour, and salt together in another bowl. Add dry ingredients alternately with milk to wet mixture. Mix to combine. Add blueberries to mixture and mix to combine. Line a muffin tin with cupcake liners and put the batter into molds about 2/3 full for each. Allow to bake for 20 minutes. Remove from heat and cool. Top with desired frosting.

Nutritional Information per Serving:
Calories: 188.6; Total Fat: 1 g; Carbs: 41.6 g; Dietary Fiber: 3.6 g; Sugars: 4.1 g; Protein: 5.3 g; Cholesterol: 0 mg; Sodium: 501.3 mg

99. Almond Flour Brownies

Yields: 12 serving
Total Time: 55 Minutes
Prep Time:10 Minutes
Cook Time: 45 Minutes

Ingredients:
- Honey (2/3 cup)
- Butter (1/2 cup, unsalted, melted)
- Vanilla Extract (1 tbsp.)
- Eggs (3)
- Almond Flour (1 cup)
- Cocoa (1/2 cup)
- Baking Soda (1/4 tsp.)
- Sea Salt (1/4 tsp.)

Directions
Set your oven to preheat to 350 degrees F, and prepare an 8x8x2-inch baking pan by lightly greasing with butter. Combine all your wet ingredients in a large bowl. Add your dry ingredients and fold until fully blended.

Tip: Consider setting batter in the refrigerator for a few minutes before cooking to allow the batter to become thicker in texture.

Pour your mixture into the prepared baking pan and set to bake until cooked (about 25 minutes, should feel like a cake). Cool, slice and serve.

Nutritional Information per Serving:
Calories: 138; Total Fat: 12.4 g; Carbs: 12 g; Dietary Fiber: 2.6 g; Sugars: 1 g; Protein: 4.2 g; Cholesterol: 61 mg; Sodium: 100 mg

100. <u>Vegan Walnut Almond Cupcakes</u>

Yields: 12 serving
Total Time: 45 Minutes
Prep Time: 10 Minutes
Cook Time: 35 Minutes

Ingredients
- Almond Flour (1 ½ cup)
- Baking soda (1 teaspoon)
- Ginger (1 tsp, ground)
- Cinnamon (1 teaspoon)
- Nutmeg (1/4 tsp)
- Salt (1/2 teaspoon)
- Coconut sugar (1 ¼ cup)
- Stevia (1/4 cup)
- Baking powder (1/2 teaspoon)
- Canola oil (1/2 cup)
- Soy yogurt (2 teaspoons, vanilla)
- Vanilla (1 teaspoon)
- Walnuts (1 cup, chopped)

Directions
Preheat the oven to 350° F. Sift baking powder, flour, baking soda, cinnamon, ginger, salt and nutmeg in a big bowl. Mix to combine. Whisk oil, stevia, coconut sugar, vanilla, and yogurt together in a different bowl. Add the liquid mixture to dry ingredients and mix to combine; try not to over mix. Put in walnuts and fold in. Line a muffin tin with paper liners and put the batter into molds about 2/3 full for each. Bake for 20 minutes and remove from heat. Allow to cool and add the desired frosting.

Nutritional Information per Serving:
Calories: 315.7; Total Fat: 27 g; Carbs: 12.3 g; Dietary Fiber: 6 g; Sugars: 1.1 g; Protein: 10.6 g; Cholesterol: 58.1 mg; Sodium: 316.6 mg

101. <u>Coconut Cupcakes</u>

Yields: 16 serving
Total Time: 50 Minutes
Prep Time: 10 Minutes
Cook Time: 40 Minutes

Ingredients
- Coconut flour (2 cups)
- Baking powder (2 teaspoons)
- Salt (1/4 teaspoon)
- Coconut (1/2 cup, flaked)
- Dairy-free soy margarine (1 stick, cold)
- Coconut sugar (1 1/3 cup)
- Coconut milk (1 cup)
- Egg Replacer powder (3 tablespoons dissolved in ¼ cup hot water)
- Apple cider vinegar (1 teaspoon)

Directions
Preheat the oven to 350° F. Sift baking powder, flour, salt and coconut in a medium bowl; combine. Mix sugar and margarine in a large bowl and use a mixer to cream until fluffy. Add egg replacer mix, coconut milk, vinegar and beat to combine.

Add dry mixture to liquid and combine. Line muffin pan with liners and put the batter in molds about 2/3 full in each. Bake for 22 minutes and remove from heat. Allow to cool and add the desired frosting.

Nutritional Information per Serving:
Calories: 324.9; Total Fat: 15.3 g; Carbs: 43.4 g; Dietary Fiber: 1.4 g; Sugars: 32.1 g; Protein: 3.7 g; Cholesterol: 51.6 mg; Sodium: 100.4 mg

101   <u>Cranberry Cupcakes</u>

Yields: 12 serving
Total Time: 40 Minutes
Prep Time: 10 Minutes
Cook Time: 30 Minutes

Ingredients
- Egg Replacer (2 tablespoons)
- Hot water (1/4 cup)
- Flour (1 ½ cups)
- Coconut sugar (3/4 cup)
- Baking powder (1 teaspoon)
- Baking soda (1/2 teaspoon)
- Salt (1/4 teaspoon)
- Cranberries (1/2 cup, with sauce)
- Dairy-free soy margarine (1/2 cup, melted)
- Dairy-free soy yogurt (1/2 cup)
- Vanilla extract (1 teaspoon)
- Nutmeg (1/2 teaspoon)

Directions
Preheat the oven to 350 degrees F. Mix egg replacer with hot water and set to the side. Sift flour, nutmeg, baking soda, sugar, salt, and baking powder in a medium bowl. Make a hole in the center of the sifted ingredients. Put the margarine, egg replacer and vanilla with each other. Combine wet ingredients together (use cranberries, reserving some of the sauce) and then mix with dry ingredients. Try not to over mix. Line muffin tin with cupcake liners and put the batter into molds about 2/3 full for each. Bake for 20 minutes and remove from heat. Drizzle with cranberry sauce, cool and top with desired frosting.

Nutritional Information per Serving:

Calories: 250; Total Fat: 11 g; Carbs: 34 g; Dietary Fiber: 1 g; Sugars: 18 g; Protein: 4 g; Cholesterol: 0.0 mg; Sodium: 280 mg

Conclusion

Congratulations on getting to the end of Ketogenic Vegetarian Cookbook. Think of this as your first Ketogenic Vegetarian hurdle, and the first of many positive hurdles to come. I hope you have enjoyed all 101-delicious ketogenic vegetarian recipes, and that you will continue to enjoy them with your whole family.

What happens next?

The next step is to continue mixing and matching these recipes as you see fit. Then when you are ready to begin another adventure join us again on another one of our other amazing culinary journeys. Remember to leave us a positive review if you liked what you read.

Until next time, keep cooking, and moving towards all your health goals. Best of luck!

Keto Bread

The Best Low Carb Backers Recipes For Ketogenic, Paleo, & Gluten Free Diets.

Written By

Denise S. Redmond

Introduction

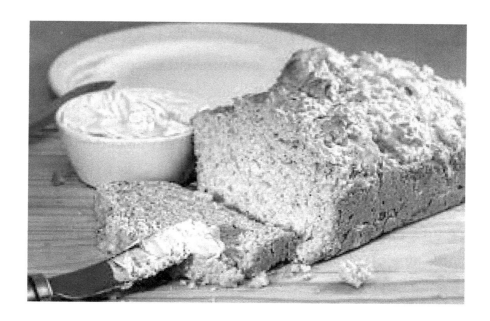

14. What exactly is a Ketogenic Diet?

Ketogenic diet was born out of "Ketosis", a process through which your body is able to break down more fat into free-fatty acid, as a result of consuming low carb diet such as Ketogenic diet. The fatty acids and ketones released as a result of this break down will produce more energy for the body.

Free fatty acids and Ketones are often released simultaneous during the breakdown of fats in the body, and with more ketones and fatty acids in the body, your body will have more energy to burn as fuel. Normally, the body burns Glucose- a produce released from the breakdown of sugar from carbohydrates (carb).

When your body burns Glucose as a form of energy, the stored fat in your body remain, but when the body burns fatty acids and Ketones when there is less sufficient glucose (as a result of consuming ketogenic diet), the body will quickly use up store fat in vital organs such as the liver, and the muscles. The overall effect of this process is that you lose weight rapidly and still find sufficient energy to sustain your daily activities.

You need to take note that, the body can only burn any energy source present, and with a low carb ketogenic diet, there is little amount of carb present, thus the body will turn to fat as a source of fuel.

When you consume high carb diet, the body burns the carbs as energy, but the fact that there is excess means the body has to store them somewhere (the muscles and organs). When excess carbs are not used up accordingly, they will make you gain more weight rapidly, especially when you are not active. With a Ketogenic diet, you feel more satisfied quickly when you eat, thus you consume much less carbs that may eventually get broken down and stored as fat in your organs and muscles. Ketogenic diet will help the body use up more stored energy. With the use up of more energy, your Insulin hormones become more regulated.

Ketogenic diet is not a magical weight loss trick, however, you should recognize that calories matter, when it comes to weight loss. In order to lose weight and remain healthy, there must be an energy balance in your body, and this balance can only be made when you use more energy than you consume. Ketogenic diet works in two ways; first it does not put you in any starving mode, secondly, it creates a net-balance in the way you ingest and use up energy.

If your body gets all it energy from the diet you ingest on daily basis, it becomes almost impossible to measure how much energy you use up, but when you are sure that your ketogenic diet has less carbs , and more of other nutrients, it is easier to detect whether you are creating a net-balance of energy. While some people eat when they are hungry, and consume what they need to become satisfied, others do eat to the fullest capacity , regardless of whether they are hungry or not. When you eat not to get full, it is easier to lose weight.

The basic principle of Ketogenic diet is that you must avoid starchy foods (most especially high carb processed foods), grains, tubers and sugars. These should be replaced with meat, leafy greens, above-ground vegetables, dairy, nuts and seeds, avocado, berries and some fats such as cream cheese and coconut oil.

Chapter 1 - Types of Ketogenic diets

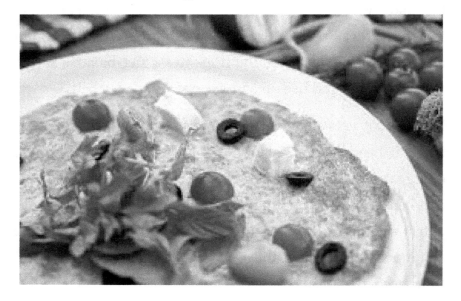

Ketogenic diet is a low carb with high fat diet, there are more than 20 recent researches that have concluded that this type of diet can actually help you lose weight steadily, on a long term. There are some researches that show the beneficial effects of Keto diets on disorders such as diabetes, Alzheimer and cancer.

No other food components have been debated like fat vs Carbs in the past few decades. According to a randomized trial of low carb diet for obesity, which was published in New England Journal of Medicine, 2003. 63 individuals were subjected to random low fat diets and low carb diets and were observed for a total of 12 months. It was observed at the end of the 12 months that the low-carb diet group lost an average of 7.3% of their body weights, while the low fat groups lost an average of 4.5% of their body weights.

The motive behind Ketogenic diet is the drastic reduction in the carb levels in meals, and this will end up putting the body into a "Ketosis" phase. Ketogenic diets share a wide range of similarities with Atkins and low carb diets but they are quite different from each other.

When your body enters the Ketosis phase as a result of continuous consumption of ketogenic diet, it becomes extremely efficient in burning fat, in order to generate energy for the body. Ketosis also speed up metabolism in the body, a situation whereby fat will be turned into Ketones in vital organs such as the liver, and that means more energy supplied to the brain.

Ketogenic diets are known to cause a massive reduction in blood sugar as well as insulin hormones supplied and with an increase production of Ketones, there are numerous benefits you can expect from consuming ketogenic diets on a regular basis.

There are several types of Ketogenic diets, however, all of them are classified into four, these are;

- The Standard Ketogenic diet (SKD)

The Standard Ketogenic diet is the commonest form of Ketogenic diet recommended for individuals who want to enjoy its maximum benefits. It comprises of a very low carb, with moderate protein and high fat diet components. The typical standard ketogenic diet comprises of 75% healthy fat, with 15% protein, 5% carb and 5% Vitamins and essential minerals.

- The Cyclical Ketogenic Diet (CKD),

The Cyclical Ketogenic Diet CKD is a special type of ketogenic diet whereby the beneficiary receives some refeeds of higher carbs for few days after taking low carb for a very long time. An example of Cyclical Ketogenic Diet is; 5 days of low carb ketogenic diet, followed by 2 days of high carb diets. This type of ketogenic diet is usually recommended for individuals suffering from certain ailments such as diabetes, and those suffering from certain nutritional disorders.

- The Targeted Ketogenic Diet (TKD),

The Targeted Ketogenic diet TKD is a special Ketogenic diet that only allows you to time your keto meals around your workouts. It is mostly recommended for those trying to speed up their weight loss or build lean muscles around specific parts of their bodies. When you target your Ketogenic diets around your workout sessions, you must have achieved a healthy weight loss and all you need is to build lean muscles. If you are overweight or obese, you need to pursue the standard Ketogenic diet.

- The High Protein Ketogenic Diet (HKD).

The High protein ketogenic diet is quite similar to the Standard ketogenic diet; however, it comes with higher protein contents. In this situation, the ratio of fat to protein and carb are; 65, 35, and 5% respectively.

It should be noted that only the Standard and high protein ketogenic diet are being investigate for their effectiveness in weight loss and general wellbeing. Cyclical and Targeted Ketogenic diets are considered to be advanced ketogenic diets that are not usually recommended for individuals trying to lose weight.

A study in the United Kingdom reveals that people indulging in Ketogenic diet are 2.5 times more likely to lose weight that those that are placed on calorie-restricted diets. It was also observed that people who consume ketogenic diets on the regular have improved lower triglycerides and cholesterols, more than individuals placed on calorie restricted diets. Another UK study shows that participants on Ketogenic diets lost three times more weight than those placed on UK special diabetes diet, which is being recommended for those suffering from diabetes and some nutritional disorder problems.

There are numerous reasons why Ketogenic diet appears to be superior to all fad diets, one of such is the increased protein, which comes with numerous health benefits, the other is the increased level of ketones which lower the total blood sugar levels which also means, an improvement in insulin sensitivity.

The bottom line on Ketogenic diet is that it speeds up your weight loss faster than low fat diet, and you don't have to starve your body to lose weight.

Chapter 2 - The Importance & Benefits of Ketogenic & Gluten-free Diets

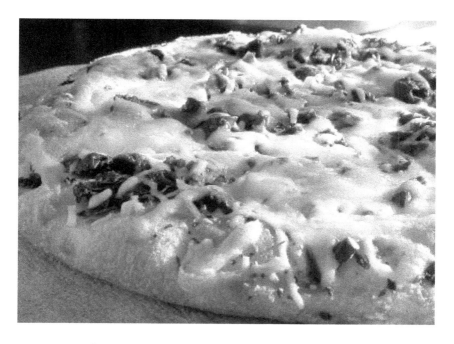

Ketogenic diet is most beneficial for overweight, as well as diabetic and pre-diabetic patients. Diabetes is a condition associated with metabolism, irregular insulin functioning, and high blood sugar. Following a ketogenic diet plan strictly can help cut down excess fat speedily, and this has been linked with type 2 diabetes, pre-diabetes and metabolic syndrome.

A study revealed how Insulin sensitivity in some groups of diabetic patients, was improved by a staggering 75%. Another study on type 2 diabetes revealed that 7 out of the 21 participants who were placed on medications, were able to stop such medications by the end of their ketogenic diet regimen.

According to a recent study on the effectiveness of Ketogenic diet on weight loss, a group of type 2 diabetic patients were found to have lost a collective weight of 24.4 lbs. or 11.1 kg, when fed with ketogenic diet for a period of time, compared to 15.2lbs. of weight loss recorded for those fed with moderate carb diets. This is an important discovery, considering the fact that excessive weight gain is linked to type 2 diabetes.

Contrary to the belief by many that Ketogenic diets will raise cholesterol levels in the body because of its low carb and high protein and fat components, the reverse is the case. Since the body will be switched to fat-burner instead of carb-reliant, the amount of fat absorbed will be too little, as long as the main source of energy is not carb but fat. Ketogenic diet forces the body to rely on fat for its primary source of energy, instead of carbs. Here are some other benefits of Ketogenic diet worth mentioning;

- **Removes sugar cravings and excessive appetite**

One of the main reasons people find it difficult to lose weight is that they can't control their appetite for food. Ketogenic diets help you control your eating habit because a diet rich in fat can be very satisfying within a short period of time. Once you start a Ketogenic diet, you will notice that sometimes, you just lose interest in eating, and this could be the most amazing part, especially when you struggle with some food addiction problems.

- **Speeds up weight loss and helps build more lean muscle**

Studies have shown that individual placed on low carb diets lose more than double the weight of those placed on low fat diet over the same period of time. One of the main reasons for this effect is that low carb dieters often find themselves getting rid of water quickly from their bodies, and the fact that a lower insulin level will force the kidney to shed excess sodium, in their bodies, thus leading to speedy loss in weight even within a short period of time. Once you reach your desired weight level, you may add a healthy carb, back to your daily calorie consumption.

- **Most fat lost during Ketogenic dieting will come from abdominal cavity**

One of the most fortunate things about Ketogenic dieting is that most of the fat lost come from the most difficult parts of the body, most especially the abdominal cavity. The way fat is stored in your body will determine how it affects your health. If most of the fat in your body are distributed in your mid-section, especially where vital organs are located, then your health is at most risk. Having excessive fat in the body can trigger insulin resistance, inflammation, and some other serious diseases, thus ketogenic diet is best for you if you struggle with fat deposit in your abdominal region.

- **Ketogenic diet reduces Triglycerides levels in the body**

Triglycerides have been linked with various heart diseases, and the main driver of triglycerides in the body are carbohydrates, especially those from simple sugars. When compared with other diets, low carb ketogenic diets will effectively reduce triglycerides by as much as 65% in the blood.

- **It increases HDL cholesterol levels in the body**

HDL cholesterol, also known a High density Lipoprotein is normally referred to good cholesterol, which is healthy for the body. They are lipoproteins that carry cholesterol around the blood while LDL or bad cholesterol are often carried from the liver to the rest of the body, where they can be reused or excreted from the body at any time. HDL carries bad cholesterol from the body and the liver thus they can be quickly removed. One of the best possible ways of increasing your blood's HDL level is to consume low carb Ketogenic diet, it lower triglyceride formation and keep your vital organs healthier.

- **Reduces blood sugar levels and regulates Insulin tolerance**

One of the greatest news for diabetes patients is that Ketogenic diets are capable of reducing blood sugar levels. When you eat high carb foods, they will be broken down into simple sugars, especially in the digestive tracts. When simple sugars enter the blood stream, they quickly raise blood sugar levels and insulin sensitivity. Healthy people will have quickly insulin regulating their blood sugar level but diabetic patients may not be as lucky and a sharp increase in sugar in the blood may cause harm.

When you develop insulin resistance, it means your body cells don't receive sufficient amount of insulin to carry blood sugar into cells but when you consume a low carb ketogenic diet, you will eliminate the need for excess insulin, and your blood sugar becomes normalized.

- **It minimizes blood pressure**

Having elevated blood pressure all the time will increase your risks to several kinds of diseases, including heart diseases, kidney failure and stroke. Low carb diets have been found through clinical researches to lower the chances of developing these diseases.

- **Low carb diets help eliminate various metabolic syndromes**

Metabolic syndromes have been linked with several other diseases such as diabetes and heart diseases. Metabolic syndromes are actually symptoms of other disorders such as ; abdominal obesity, high blood pressure, high blood sugar levels, and High triglycerides. The good news is that low carb diet will greatly improve these symptoms once you start taking ketogenic diets.

- **Provides therapeutic effects for many brain disorders**

Though, Glucose is necessary for a healthy and functional brain, but some parts of the brain can only burn glucose and when we do not eat sufficient carbs, the liver will produce more glucose from protein. Some parts of the brain also burn ketones, especially when you are in a starving mode or when you consume low carb diets. Ketogenic diets have been used for decades to help kids suffering from epilepsy and when they are not responding to conventional treatments.

- **Boosts immunity**

The overall conclusion of consuming low carb diets is that the immunity of the whole system is strengthened against harmful diseases.

Chapter 3 – What to Eat & Avoid on the Keto Diet

Foods to Avoid				
Sweet Fruits	Soda & Carbonated Drinks	Fruit Juice Concentra rates	Sugary Smoothies	Processed sugars
Processed Pasta, Flours & Related Products	Any Breads that is Not a Keto Bread	Sugary condiments	Sugary Candies	Sugary Ice Creams
Root Vegetables	Processed Rice	**All Alcoholic Beverages**	**Hydrogenated Oils**	**Saturated & Unhealthy Fats**

Foods to Enjoy

Steak	Ham	Sausage	Lean Meat	Mackerel	Salmon
		Poultry			Tuna
		Turkey	Bacon	Sardines	
Eggs	Tout	Organic Salads	Creamy Salads	Unprocessed Blue Cheese	Unprocessed Cream Cheese
Unprocessed	Unprocessed	Unprocessed Mozzare	Walnuts	Flaxseeds	Coconut Oil

Goat Cheese	Cheddar Cheese	lla Cheese			
Almonds	Pumpkin Seeds	Chia Seeds	Extra Virgin Olive Oil	Avocado Oil	Low Carb Vegetables
Salt	Pepper	Herbs	Spices	Berries in Moderation	

Chapter 4 - Ketogenic

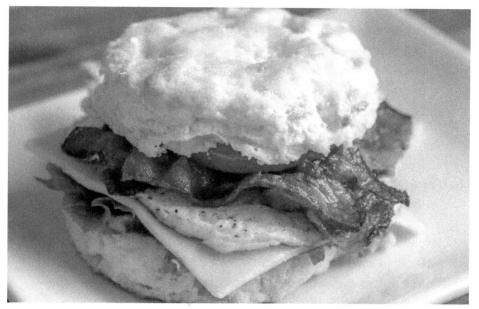

Diet Protocols

Ketogenic diet protocol or rules dictates the right amount of each food (maximum), that must be included at a time in your meals. It also explains how to make your choices and adhere to the low carb principles of the diet.

Here are Ketogenic diet protocols you need to follow;

15. Animal Foods
- Meat and fish provide 0-net carbs and must not exceed 150g/ serving
- Eggs provide about 1.4 net carbs (grams), this must not exceed 150g per serving,
- Full fat cream provides 1.6 net carb, it must not exceed ¼ a cup or 60ml per serving.
- Cheese (hard), provides 0.4 net carb and must not exceed 30g per serving.
- Cream cheese (full fat), provides 1.6 net carbs, and must not exceed ¼ cup or 50g per serving.

16. Vegetables
- Vegetables such as Lettuce, Asparagus, Cucumber, Cooked spinach, Cabbage, Celery stalk, Cauliflower, Chopped Broccoli, and Dark leaf kale provides between 1.2 and 6.4 net carb (grams) and should not exceed 150g per serving.
- Vegetables such as Brown or white mushrooms, Onions Tomatoes, green or red pepper, green beans, garlic and white slice onions provide between 1.2 and 5.9 net calories(grams) , these should not exceed ½ cup or 50grams per serving.

17. Fruits
- Sliced strawberries produce up to 4.7(grams) and should not exceed ½ a cup or 85g per serving.
- Raspberries produce about 3.3 net carbs, and must not exceed ½ a cup or 62g per serving.
- Blackberries provide some 3.2 net carbs and must not exceed ½ a cup or 72 grams per serving.
- Blueberries contain some 8.9 net carbs, and must not exceed ½ a cup or 74g per serving.
- Avocado provides about 3.7 net carbs and should be pierced into an average of 200g per serving.

18. Nuts and seeds
- Almonds provide about 2.7 net carbs (grams), and should not exceed 30g per serving.
- Hazelnuts provide about 2 net carbs (grams) and should not exceed 30g per serving.
- Walnuts provides some 2 net carbs (grams), and should not exceed 30g per serving.
- Other seeds such as Chia seeds, sunflower seeds, Pumpkin seeds, and pecans provide between 0.4 and 7.6 net carbs (grams), and should not exceed a tablespoon or 30g per serving.

19. Condiments and spices
- Condiments, sauce and other related extras such as unsweetened Almond milk, creamed coconut milk, olive oil, mustard, tomato puree, apple cider vinegar, dark chocolate, flax meal, stevia, dry red or white wine, provides between 0.1 and 5.7 net carbs, and must not be included at levels of between ¼ cup (60mls), and 1 glass per serving.

20. Fish, Meat, and Sea foods-protocol
- You should consider eating a fish that was caught, these include; Cod, Flounder, Halibut, tuna, Salmon, Trout, and mackerel. Shellfishes you can consume include ; Scallops, Lobsters, Clams, Crab, mussels and squids. Fishes can make up the bulk of your diet and it is recommended that you consume not less than 250g per serving.
- Meat such as Veal, beef, goat, wild game and any organically fed animal are the best because they contain higher fatty acid count. This should be primary component of your Ketogenic diet and must be included at not less than 400g a day.

- Pork may be included or alternated with meat and fish. You should aim at Pork chops, pork loins, and ham (try as much as possible to avoid any added sugar to the ham). Pork should be included in your diet at not more than 150g at a time.
- Bacon and sausage are ideal, but try as much as possible to avoid any added sugars in the ham. Bacon and sausage should be added at not more than 100g per serving.
- Peanut butter- Natural peanut butter is the best but you need to exercise caution because they contain high amount of omega 6 and carbs. An ideal option is Macadamia nut butter. Peanut butter should be sparingly used in any Ketogenic diet.

21. General Ketogenic diet protocol
- The general protocol of Ketogenic dieting is that a minimum of 80% of your diet should comprise of healthy fat, while 15% should contain essential proteins, vitamins and minerals. Any Ketogenic diet must contain less than 5 % of carbs, because you want to cut down on carbohydrates and force your body to burn more fat as energy.
- Depending on the duration you want to go, it is ideal to start with a 72-hour Ketogenic diet straight, whereby you have a day or 2 to prepare your body and then start the Ketogenic diet on the third day through to the fifth day. One of the benefits of having a gradual Ketogenic diet regimen is that it helps your body recover quickly from any effect that might result from enforcing Ketogenic diets and getting a break after each 3 days is the best possible way of achieving this.
- Try as much as possible to substitute the foods in each recommended category, to ensure that you don't get bored eating the same food all the time. For instance, you can consume fish and pork today, then consume more of beef and chicken the following day.

- Being active during your Ketogenic diet regimen is recommended, however, you don't have to be involved in high impact exercises. A moderate impact exercise is recommended to help you burn fat. The most effective exercises for Ketogenic diet are performed very early in the morning, before 7AM and late in the evening, around 6-7PM. Low impact exercises recommended for Ketogenic diet regimen include; stretching exercises, cardio workouts, weight lifting, aerobics, cycling, swimming and brisk walking.

Chapter 5 - Baking Keto Bread

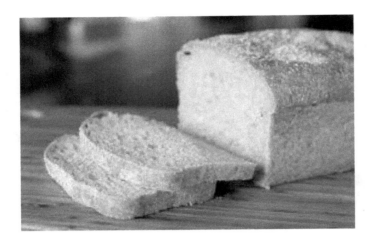

There are several methods of baking Keto bread, the most prominent among these are:

22. The Straight Dough Method

In this case, all the ingredients needed for the kept bread are mixed together before the dough is fermented over a period of time. The strength of the flour should determine the fermentation time, generally, stronger flours will require longer fermentation time, and hence it will take longer time to mature properly. It should be noted that flours that will require between 2 and 3 hours to mature should be used in the making of keto bread, and by straight method.

Flours that take more than 3 hours to mature, should not be used in the making of keto bread because the temperature of the dough becomes hard to monitor during the long fermentation periods. Extreme rise in temperature of the dough may trigger an acidic taste and flavor.

23. The No Time Dough Method

This method usually involves the dough being fermented in some unusual manner. In this case, the dough is only allowed to ferment for about 30 minutes and the reason being that it needs to recover quickly from the strains applied during mixing. Since the dough is probably not fermented in this case, additional yeast (2-3 times higher than usually quantities), is added to compensate for the production of gas and conditioning of the dough. The No Time Dough method of baking keto bread is usually done during emergencies, however bread, made through this method usually have poor shelf life.

Due to the absence of fermentation, the dough wouldn't be conditioned properly, in order for better moisture retention.

24. The Salt Delay Method

This method is suitable for those who want to lose weight and at the same time control their salt intake. This method is a slight variation of the Straight Dough Method of baking. In this situation, all the ingredients are mixed together except the salt, and fat. It is believed that addition of the salt will make it have some control over the enzymatic action over the yeast. Fermentation through a salt delay method in dough making, will be faster, hence this method of keto bread making is often preferred.

For Keto bread making, less than half of the usual salt should be added at a knock-back phase of the dough making. The salt should be sifted into the dough, or it may be creamed with fat. The Keto bread dough should be free of gluten; hence it should take a shorter time for the dough to set.

25. The Sponge & Dough Method
This method was designed based on the fact that stronger flour will take too long to condition, hence the straight dough method should not be used in making keto bread because the fermentation will take a shorter time. For such strong flours, a Sponge and dough method will be more suitable because the method helps where the issue of improper control of dough temperature sets in.

To make a Keto bread through a Sponge and dough method, you need your Keto flour (very low in non-processed components, and carb), the appropriate amount of water, yeast, and brown sugar, all mixed together. Longer fermentation in Sponge and dough method will allow the dough to mix properly. The sponge is fermented for a pre-determined period of time, and in most cases, it may take up to 16 hours for the fermentation to be completed. The flexibility of this method of making keto bread dough makes it suitable because there is an increased flavor of the final bread, brought about by longer hours of fermentation.

Another benefit of using the sponge and dough method to make keto bread is that less yeast will be needed because the yeast will multiply rapidly during the sponge fermenting process.

26. The Ferment & Dough Method

This method is a type of variation to the sponge and dough method. The keto bread made from this dough making will normally contain eggs, milk, and some fat, however, brown sugar must still be used. It is believed that the addition of all those ingredients will retard the activities of the yeast. When all ingredients are mixed perfectly, the yeast will get a conducive environment that will make it more aggressive.

The fermentation time in the Ferment and dough method of making dough should depend on preference of the dough maker, and the type of final bread product. It should be noted that a fermenting dough with milk, may cause the production of more lactic acid- though this does not affect the final carb composition of the keto bread, but the final flavor taste and texture may be negatively affected.

Chapter 6 -Errors to Avoid on a Keto Diet

You need to pay careful attention to certain things, if you truly want to achieve sustainable, long term weight loss through the consumption of Ketogenic diets, especially Keto breads.

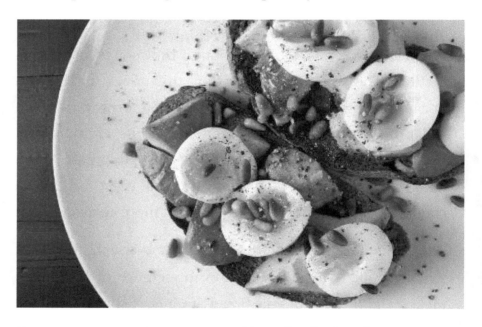

Error #1: Ignoring your sodium body levels

One of the most prominent mistakes among individuals who consume Ketogenic diets is that they tend to ignore the fact that they need to replenish their body's sodium levels. One of the benefits of Ketogenic diets is that they normalize your body's insulin levels, therefore your body will not become resistance to the hormones- (insulin resistance can trigger diabetes and some other blood sugar problems).

One of the main functions of Insulin hormones is to instruct fat cells to store nutrients, likewise, it enforces the Kidney to retain more sodium minerals in the body. Shortage of Insulin hormones means your kidneys wouldn't store as much Sodium as it used to. Aside Sodium minerals, your body will also shed substantial amount of water within the first 24 hours of consuming Ketogenic diet, a condition that can help you get rid of bloating.

Your body needs substantial amount of sodium, the shedding of sodium continuously through Ketogenic diets may result in slight side effects such as light-headedness, fatigue, constipation and headache. The best possible way of avoiding this problem is to increase your salt intake slightly, but not too much to cause overload of sodium.

For your Keto bread, you need to add a substantial amount of salt (½ to 2 teaspoons of table salt is required when mixing the keto bread dough)

Error #2: Consuming too much Protein in your Ketogenic diets

The second most prominent error many ketogenic diet eaters make is that they replace most of their carbs with protein, instead of healthy fats. Your body will not enter Ketogenesis with high protein contents, even though protein is an essential component of healthy diets and it increases satiety, making you get fuller quickly. When you consume more lean proteins, the excess will be converted into glucose, which means your body will not produce enough ketosis and fatty acids to turn it into fat-burning mode. Proteins should not exceed 20% of the total Ketogenic diet, while carbs should be less than 6%.

Error #3: Eating more carbs than the recommended levels

Ideally, you should aim at 5% carbs in your Ketogenic meals, when you consume up to 10% carbs, your body may find it extremely hard to enter the Ketogenic mode. In the beginning of Ketogenic diet consumption, most people get confused about what constitutes a 5% carb in their meals, many may believe that anything less than 120-150g of car, is "low carb". You may not have any problem entering Ketogenic phase when you consume 150g of carbs from unprocessed foods, however, carbonated sugary drinks, overripe fruits, and starchy foods can rapidly increase your carb intake , thus forcing you to break the Ketogenic diet rule on carbs. Sugary foods can lead to a spike in blood sugar, a situation that can trigger more secretion of Insulin hormones, thus making it impossible to attain a Ketogenic phase. It may take some home experiments before you learn to make accurate measurement of your carbs, but experts suggest that you should stick within the 50-100g of carbs a day, from healthy and unprocessed foods.

Error #4: Lack of patience

You should keep in mind that Ketogenic diet is not a quick solution to weight loss problems, rather it takes a gradual, steady and long-term approach to speed up fat-burning process. In addition to this, the diet plan will require some amounts of dedication and consistencies, to make it work. Many Ketogenic diet users often run into a stumbling block, when they expect too much from this weight loss therapy within the shortest period of time, with some even trying to starve themselves – starvation will only yield a temporary weight loss result, while Ketogenic diets produce long term, sustainable weight loss.

The body is conditioned to burn carbs, until you force it to burn fat through Ketogenic weight loss. Drastically reducing your carb intake, may take a while to achieve, and until you reach the desirable low carb intake, your body will not enter Ketogenic phase. The full adaptation of your body to Ketogenic phase may take between few days and weeks, hence you have to be patient to see the best possible results.

Error #5: You are scared of eating fat

Media propaganda against fat has forced many away from Ketogenic diets, but the revelation of more truth about saturated fats, through Ketogenic diets has proven that switching the body from carb-reliant to fat-burning mode, is the best sustainable way to lose weight steadily with little or no side effects. Eating Ketogenic diets does not mean you must consume all kinds of fats, you still need to avoid bad cholesterol, especially those found in hydrogenated vegetable oils, and fast-foods, that are known to increase the risks of inflammation and several diseases. You should aim at replacing fats such as vegetable oils with bacon grease and coconut oil.

Error #6: Trying to enforce too many changes on yourself, at once

Changing some addictive lifestyles such as excessive alcohol consumption, smoking, consumption of sweetened beverages and sedentary lifestyles, can be very challenging for most people who want to enjoy the benefits of Ketogenic diet. There should be a period where your body must be prepared for switching to Ketogenic diet. Taking an abrupt approach to changing your lifestyle may trigger certain withdrawal symptoms , for instance, withdrawal from smoking abruptly may trigger some symptoms such as migraine headaches, lack of sleep, persistent coughing and sharp increase in appetite. You need to take a gradual approach by cutting your smoking habits, and alcohol consumption and then take on a low-impact daily exercise, to ensure that your body adjusts perfectly when you eventually introduce Ketogenic diet plans.

Individuals who make adequate preparation before venturing into Ketogenic dieting for weight loss, will end up with more positive results than those who do not prepare themselves enough.

Error #7: Not matching your Ketogenic diets properly

A slight break of Ketogenic diet protocol may affect the results you get on the long run. You need to mix and match your diet components in such a way that none of the Ketogenic diet protocols is broken. You can achieve this by creating a timetable where similar food components can be substituted with each other, and unhealthy items can be replaced with healthier substitutes. You should alternate between similar foods, to ensure that you don't get bored quickly, likewise you must stay hydrated, to ensure that your body retains more fluid. Don't be discouraged if you break the Ketogenic diet protocols, once in a while, you can always continue from that point, until you master such rules.

Chapter 7 - Keto bread, muffins, Waffles, Bagels and others

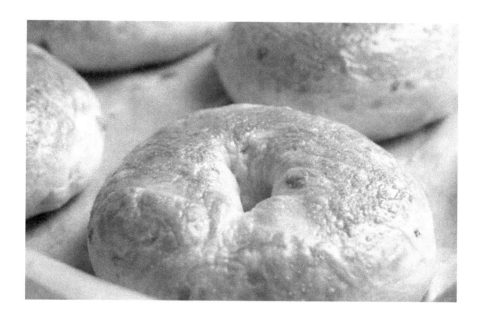

The delicious recipes featured in this chapter would be the perfect for those of us who love breads, waffles and sandwiches but not sure how to incorporate healthier types of breads while maintaining your Ketogenic nutritional daily requirements.

Thank you for allowing us to expose you to the large variety of Keto Bread recipes that you can enjoy, please feel free to leave us a positive review if you like what you are about to read through.

1. KETO BANANA LOAF

Yield: 3 Servings

Total Time: 1 Hour 20 Minutes

Prep Time: 20 Minutes

Cook Time: 1 Hour

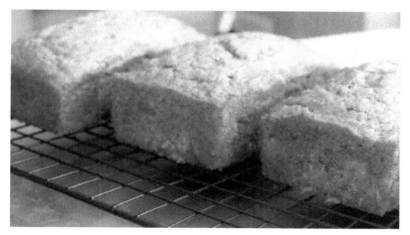

Ingredients:

- 12 ounces of soft cream cheese,
- 5 large eggs,
- A cup of mashed 3 large bananas,
- ½ cup of soy protein powder,
- A teaspoon of baking powder,
- A teaspoon of baking powder,
- 4 teaspoons of Splenda (sugar substitute),
- 2 teaspoons of grated lemon peel,
- A cup of unprocessed wheat bran, and
- A cup of whole almond meal.

Directions:

Pre-heat the oven to about 325 degree F, and then butter lightly, the mini loaf pans. Cut some strips of waxed paper to fit the bottoms of the pan, and allow them to hang over the edges. Get the cream cheese and eggs in the electric mixer bowl, and beat until flat. Add the remaining eggs (one at a time), add all other ingredients and then beat at a slow speed. Add the nuts and bran and spoon the batter into the pans. Bake the bread for about an hour until done and serve immediately.

Nutritional Information per Serving:

Calories: 269; Total Fat: 22 g; Carbs: 15 g; Dietary Fiber: 4 g;
Protein: 8 g; Cholesterol: 63 mg; Sodium: 147 mg

2. KETOGENIC OOPSIE BREAD ROLLS

Yield: 6 Servings

Total Time: 1 Hour

Prep Time: 20 Minutes

Cook Time: 40 Minutes

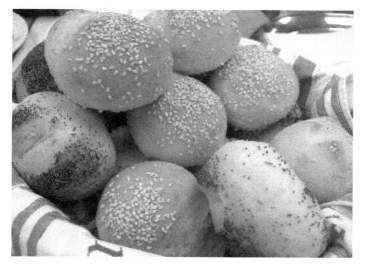

Ingredients:

- 3 medium to large eggs,
- Non-sticky cooking spray,
- 1/8 teaspoon of tartar cream,
- 2 ½ ounces of full-fat cold cubed cream cheese,
- 1/6 teaspoon of salt.

Directions:

Pre-heat the oven to about 300-degree F, then line some cookie sheet with parchment paper, before spraying with cooking spray. Separate the eggs, and avoid mixing the yolk with the egg whites, and then place the egg white inside a clean bowl. With the aid of a clean non-greasy electric whisk, simply whisk the egg white with the tartar cream until the mix becomes stiff.

Get a separate bowl and inside make use of the same whisk to mix together the yolk, salt, and cream cheese, until the mix is perfectly smooth. With the aid of a spatula or spoon, gently fold the egg whites into the cream cheese mix, and make sure you work on batches- place a mound of egg whites at the top of the yolk mix, and then fold the yolk mix gently from underneath. And on top of the egg white, while rotating the bowl, again and again until the mixture has been perfectly incorporated. Make use of the folding technique in order to ensure that the air bubbles remain intact inside the egg white.

Spoon 6 large mounds of the mix onto the already prepared baking sheet, and gently press the spoon or spatula on top of each of the mound to flatten it slightly. Bake the bread rolls for between 30 and 40 minutes until they turn golden brown, then cool the rolls for some minutes on cooking sheet, and before transferring them unto wire rack. You may want to store leftovers inside a Ziploc bag in the fridge.

Nutritional Information per Serving:

Calories: 103; Total Fat: 9 g; Carbs: 1 g; Dietary Fiber: 1 g; Protein: 4 g; Cholesterol: 13 mg; Sodium: 10 mg

3. LOW CARB COCONUT FLOUR FLATBREAD

Yield: 2 Servings

Total Time: 1 Hour

Prep Time: 30 Minutes

Cook Time: 30 Minutes

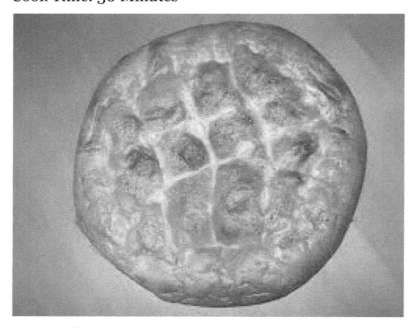

Ingredients:

- 1 medium to large egg,
- 1 teaspoon of coconut flour,
- Optional 1 teaspoon of Parmesan cheese,
- 1/8 teaspoon of baking soda,
- 1/8 teaspoon of baking powder,
- Tablespoon of butter.
- 2 pinches of salt, and

- 2 tablespoons of milk.

Directions:

Add all the ingredients and stir them until there are no lumps, let the batter sit for about a minute and you will notice it getting fluffier. Melt the butter, inside the pan before pouring 2 small size sandwich-size pancakes unto the pan. Place the pan on medium heat and when the top starts to bubble, simply flip the mix over. Put the cheese alongside the other contents on a slice, before putting the second flat bread on top. Butter both flat bread pieces before you flip it. Flip the sandwich flat bread when the bottom is turning brown and continue cooking until the cheese has completely melted.

Nutritional Information per Serving:

Calories: 193; Total Fat: 16 g; Carbs: 1 g; Dietary Fiber: 2 g; Protein: 6 g; Cholesterol: 0 mg; Sodium: 5 mg

4. GLUTEN-FREE COCONUT AND ALMOND BREAD

Yield: 8 Servings

Total Time: 1 Hour

Prep Time: 30 Minutes

Cook Time: 30 Minutes

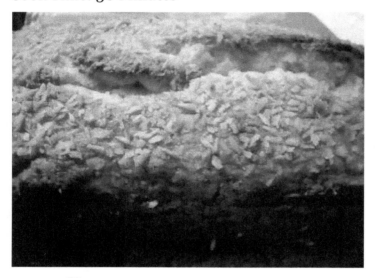

Ingredients:

- 1 3/4 of almond flour
- 1 ½ tablespoons of coconut flour
- ¼ of a cup of ground flaxseed
- ¼ tablespoon of salt
- 1 teaspoon of baking soda
- 4-5 large eggs
- ¼ of a cup of coconut oil
- 1 teaspoon of a natural sweetener such as stevia
- 1 tablespoon of apple cider vinegar

Directions:

Pre-heat the oven to about 350-degree F, and then grease the loaf of pan. Mix the almond, and coconut flour, alongside the flaxseed, salt, and baking soda, inside a food processor. Pulse the ingredients together, before you add the eggs, vinegar and oil. Pour the mix or batter inside the loaf pan, and bake for about 30 minutes at the 350-degree F in the oven. Let the bread cool for few minutes before serving.

Nutritional Information per Serving:

Calories: 193; Total Fat: 16 g; Carbs: 1 g; Dietary Fiber: 2 g; Protein: 6 g; Cholesterol: 0 mg; Sodium 10 mg

5. KETOGENIC FOCACCIA FLAX BREAD

Yield: 12 Servings

Total Time: 1 Hour

Prep Time: 30 Minutes

Cook Time: 30 Minutes

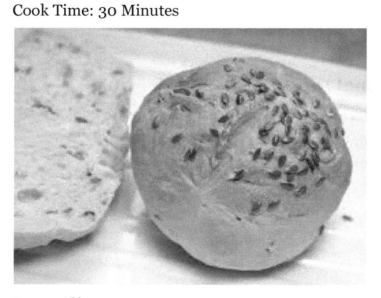

Ingredients

- 2 ½ cups of flax seed meal,
- 1 ½ teaspoons of baking powder,
- 1 teaspoon of salt,
- 1 teaspoon of brown sugar,
- 5 large beaten eggs,
- ½ a cup of water, and
- 1/3 cup of olive oil.

Directions:

Pre-heat the oven to about 350-degree F, then prepare a 10 x 15" baking pan alongside oiled parchment paper. Mix all the dry ingredients perfectly (whisk them properly). Add all the wet ingredients to the dry ingredients, and mix thoroughly, and make sure there are no strings of egg white protruding through the batter. Let the batter remain set for about 3 minutes to allow it thicken but don't leave it set for too long so that it wouldn't become too thick to spread.

Pour the batter inside the baking pan, and consider the fact that it will mound up from the middle, for this reason, you need to spread the batter away from the center, in order to achieve an even thickness inside the rectangular pan. Bake the batter for about 30
minutes until the bread springs up when you press the middle down with your finger. The bread should be turning brown once the flax meal has been perfectly cooked.   Cool the bread and slice into the appropriate sizes. You can cut through the bed with the aid of a spoon or spatula.

Nutritional Information per Serving:

Calories: 140; Total Fat: 20.5 g; Carbs: 7 g; Dietary Fiber: 4 g;
Protein: 14 g; Cholesterol: 0 mg; Sodium: 170 mg

6.SWEDISH KETO BUNS

Yield: 4 Servings

Total Time: 1 Hour

Prep Time: 25 Minutes

Cook Time: 35 Minutes

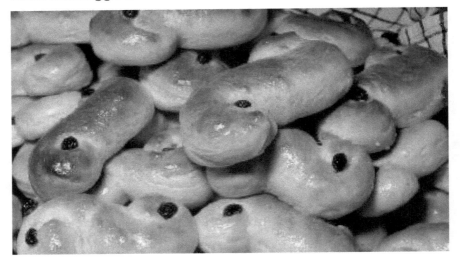

Ingredients:

- ½ a cup of almond flour,
- 1 tablespoon of whole flax seeds,
- 1 tablespoon of shelled sunflower seeds,
- 2 tablespoons of Psyllium husk power,
- 1 tablespoon of baking powder,
- ½ a teaspoon of salt,
- 2 tablespoons of extra virgin olive oil,
- 2 large eggs, and
- ½ cup of sour cream

Directions:

Pre-heat the oven to about 400 degree F, Mix the almond flour with the seeds salt, Psyllium, and baking powder inside a medium to large bowl. Add the eggs, olive oil, and sour cream and mix gently for about 2 minutes. Let the mi sit for about 5 minutes.

Cut the dough into 4 and then shape them into balls before putting them inside a cake pan and make sure you use parchment papers to prevent sticking. Bake the buns for about 25 minutes until they turn brown and serve when hot.

Nutritional Information per Serving:

Calories: 120; Total Fat: 18 g; Carbs: 4.5 g; Dietary Fiber: 2.8 g;

Protein: 12 g; Cholesterol: 0 mg; Sodium: 100 mg

7. KETO BACON MUFFINS

Yield: 12 Servings

Total Time: 1 Hour

Prep Time: 40 Minutes

Cook Time: 20 Minutes

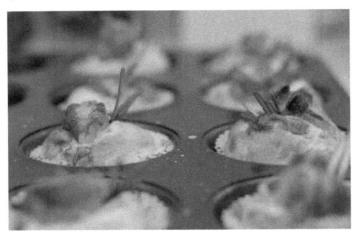

Ingredients:

- 6 fried crisps of bacon slices,
- 2/3 cup of olive oil,
- ½ cup of water,
- 1/3 cup of a whipping cream,
- 3 large eggs,
- Teaspoon of vanilla extract,
- 1 cup of vanilla whey protein powder,
- 2 teaspoons of oat flour,
- 2 teaspoons of baking powder.

Direction:

Pre-heat the oven to 350 degree F. combine the vanilla extract, eggs, and vanilla extract, mix very well before adding the whey protein powder, baking powder and oat flour. Mix until perfectly moistened, then break the bacon into small bits, before stirring into batter. Grease the muffin tins before pouring the batter into them. Bake for about 15 minutes and cool immediately. Serve after few minutes.

Nutritional Information per Serving:

Calories: 217; Total Fat: 19 g; Carbs: 3 g; Dietary Fiber: 3 g; Protein: 7 g; Cholesterol: 0 mg; Sodium: 0 mg

8. KETO BELGIAN WAFFLES

Yield: 3 Servings

Total Time: 1 Hour

Prep Time: 30 Minutes

Cook Time: 30 Minutes

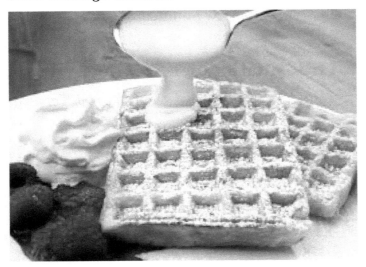

Ingredients:

- 4 tablespoons of unsalted butter,
- 4 separated large eggs,
- ¼ cup of oat flour,
- A cup of sour cream,
- ½ teaspoon of vanilla extract,
- ½ teaspoon of salt, and
- Optional 2 teaspoon of grated nutmeg.

Directions:

With the aid of electric mixer, beat the eggs, and set it aside in a bowl. In the mixer bowl, simply cream the butter, and beat-in the egg yolk. Add the flour and the sour cream, then stir in the vanilla, salt and nutmeg. Fold-in the egg whites, and then pour into a pre-heated waffle iron and bake for about 30 minutes.

Nutritional Information per Serving:

Calories: 269; Total Fat: 22 g; Carbs: 15 g; Dietary Fiber: 4 g;

Protein: 8 g; Cholesterol: 63 mg; Sodium: 147 mg

9.KETO FRENCH TOAST

Yield: 1 Serving

Total Time: 10 Minutes

Prep Time: 2 Minutes

Cook Time: 8 Minutes

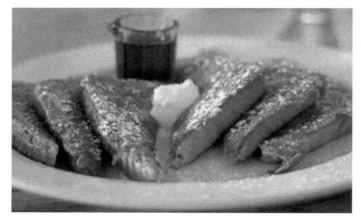

Ingredients:

- One 7 ½ inches round waffle,
- 2 large eggs,
- 2 tablespoons of light cream, and
- A tablespoon of butter.

Directions:

Gently beat the eggs, and the cream, then pour the mix in a pan that is capable of holding the waffle. Turn the waffle up to 3 times, to allow it absorb the eggs. Heat a large skillet over medium heat, and melt the butter, then add the waffle when the butter foams. Cook the waffle gently on a side until the egg is cooked, turn to the other side and cook slowly, then serve immediately with low carb syrup.

Nutritional Information per Serving:

Calories: 269; Total Fat: 22 g; Carbs: 15 g; Dietary Fiber: 4 g;

Protein: 8 g; Cholesterol: 63 mg; Sodium: 147 mg

10. KETO EGG MUFFINS RECIPE

Yield: 2-3 Servings

Total Time: 30 Minutes

Prep Time: 15 Minutes

Cook Time: 15 Minutes

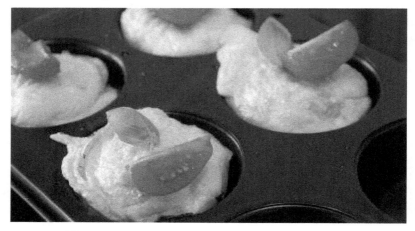

Ingredients:

- a handful of chopped vegetables (preferably, leafy green veggies)
- 1g of lean meat (this could be beef, chicken, lamb or turkey), and
- 2-3 medium to extra-large eggs.

Directions:

Chopped the leafy veggies, and add them to the lean meat and pour the mix into a non-sticky muffin pan. Whisk the egg and pour it over the top of the meat and veggies, before baking the mi in the oven until about 350 degrees until it turns brown.

You may increase the quantities of these recipes and prepare a large batch that can be re-heated when needed.

Nutritional Information per Serving:

Calories: 217; Total Fat: 19 g; Carbs: 3 g; Dietary Fiber: 3 g; Protein: 7 g; Cholesterol: 0 mg; Sodium: 0 mg

11. KETO WHOLE GRAIN FRUIT AND NUT MUFFINS

Yield: 12 Servings

Total Time: 35 Minutes

Prep Time: 20 Minutes

Cook Time: 15 Minutes

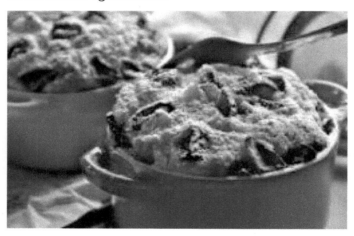

Ingredients:

- ¾ cup of gluten-free baking mix,
- ¾ cup of whole grain flour,
- 2 teaspoon of baking powder,
- ½ teaspoon of baking soda,
- ½ teaspoon of salt,
- 2 medium-large eggs,
- ¾ cup of brown sugar,
- ¾ cup of low-fat butter milk,
- ½ teaspoon of vanilla extract,
- 1 ½ cups of chopped fresh fruits, and
- 1 ½ cup of frozen berries.

Direction:

Pre-heat the oven to about 350 degrees, and coat your muffin cups with cooking spray. Whish the gluten-free mix, then whisk the egg, sugar, butter milk and vanilla in a separate bowl. Stir these in the mix and fold it in the fresh fruits and nuts. Scoop the batter inside the muffin cups and bake for about 15 minutes. Cool immediately and serve.

Nutritional Information per Serving:

Calories: 217; Total Fat: 19 g; Carbs: 3 g; Dietary Fiber: 3 g; Protein: 7 g; Cholesterol: 0 mg; Sodium: 0 mg

12. *KETO COOKIE ROLLS*

Yield: 2-3 Servings

Total Time: 1 Hour

Prep Time: 25 Minutes

Cook Time: 35 Minutes

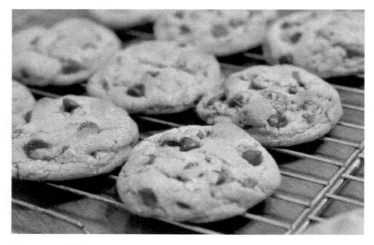

Ingredients:

- 3 eggs
- A packet of Splenda
- A dash of salt
- A pinch of cream
- 3 tablespoons of cream cheese

Directions:

Pre-heat the oven to 300 degrees F, separate the eggs and add the Splenda, cream cheese, and salt to the egg yolk. whisk the mix, then get a separate bowl, and whip the egg whites, and cream, until very stiff, then use a spatula to fold the egg yolk mix into the egg white mix(don't break down the egg white mix). Spray the cookie sheet and spoon the mix into it, then make 6 mounds, then flatten the mounds before baking for about 35 minutes, let the baked food cool for few minutes, then remove and cool.

Nutritional Information per Serving:

Calories: 269; Total Fat: 22 g; Carbs: 15 g; Dietary Fiber: 4 g;
Protein: 8 g; Cholesterol: 63 mg; Sodium: 147 mg

13. KETOGENIC DOTTIES WASSA CRACKERS

Yield: 6 Servings

Total Time: 1 Hour

Prep Time: 40 Minutes

Cook Time: 20 Minutes

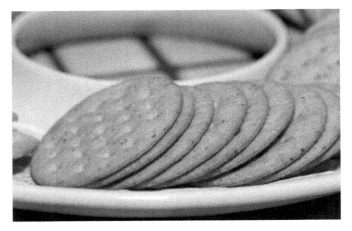

Ingredients:

- 1 cup of wheat bran,
- 2 tablespoons of oat flour,
- 2 tablespoons of whey powder,
- A tablespoon of sesame seeds,
- A teaspoon of salt, and
- 1 cup of water.

Directions:

Pre-heat the oven to about 350 degree F, spray the cookie sheet, then mix all ingredients and pour them unto the sheet-make sure the mix is spread evenly. Bake for about 10 minutes and remove the sheet from oven, score the crackers and return them into the oven. Bake further for 15 minutes. Turn off the oven and let the baked crackers settle down for about 1 hour, remove again and turn the oven to 250 degrees. Turn the crackers over with a spatula, and return them to oven and bake for about 15 minutes. Cool the crackers and serve immediately.

Nutritional Information per Serving:

Calories: 269; Total Fat: 22 g; Carbs: 15 g; Dietary Fiber: 4 g;
Protein: 8 g; Cholesterol: 63 mg; Sodium: 147 mg

14. KETOGENIC OMELET

Yield: 4 Servings

Total Time: 20 Minutes

Prep Time: 10 Minutes

Cook Time: 10 Minutes

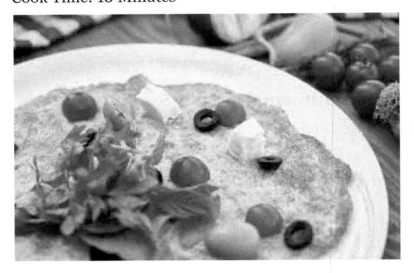

Ingredients:

- 4-5 sprays of rapeseed oil
- 30g of halved cherry tomatoes
- ¼ red onion (peeled and finely diced)
- 6 fresh basil leaves
- 2 medium or small organic eggs
- a tablespoon of grated Parmesan cheese
- Salt and pepper

Directions:

Gently heat a small non-sticky pan over heat and spray the oil inside, add the onions and fry over gentle heat for 4 minutes until they become soft. Add the cherry tomatoes and cook for further 4 minutes, until their juices are being released. Put off the heat and then add the basil leaves, and then spoon the tomato mixture inside a bowl and clean the frying pan. Beat the eggs with some little water before seasoning with salt and pepper, then heat the non-stick pan over medium heat before adding the eggs.

Swirl the eggs around the pan while you tip the pan and drawing the edges of the egg into the middle in order to allow the eggs run and set. Sprinkle the parmesan cheese on the egg when they are about to set, and then spoon the tomatoes on top of the cheese. And then cook for about 2 minutes for the omelet to set. Slide the omelet out of the pan and you may add some black pepper to season further. You can serve this meal with salad leaves.

Nutritional Information per Serving:

Calories: 269; Total Fat: 22 g; Carbs: 15 g; Dietary Fiber: 4 g;

Protein: 8 g; Cholesterol: 63 mg; Sodium: 147 mg

15. KETO BREAD RECIPE

Yield: 6 Servings

Total Time: 1 Hour

Prep Time: 20 Minutes

Cook Time: 40 Minutes

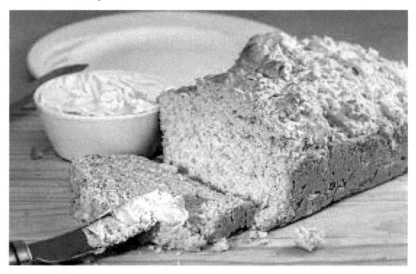

Ingredients

- 6 medium to large eggs (stored at room temperature),
- 1 cup of sifted coconut flour,
- ½ a cup of flaxseed meal,
- 1 teaspoon of salt,
- 1 teaspoon of baking powder,
- ½ teaspoon of baking soda,
- ¾ a cup of water, and
- 1 tablespoon of apple cider vinegar.

Directions:

Pre-heat the oven to about 350-degree F, and grease the baking pans before sifting the coconut flour oil inside the pan. Add all the remaining dry ingredients and whisk together inside the pan. Add the vinegar, water and eggs. Stir the mix until the batter has formed together. Bake the batter for about 40 minutes until the bread has been cooked through. Allow the bread to cool inside the baking pan until it becomes warm, then remove from the pan and slice into equal parts and serve.

Nutritional Information per Serving:

Calories: 269; Total Fat: 22 g; Carbs: 15 g; Dietary Fiber: 4 g;
Protein: 8 g; Cholesterol: 63 mg; Sodium: 147 mg

16. KETO PIZZA

Yield: 6 Servings

Total Time: 5 Hours 25 Minutes

Prep Time: 5 Hours

Cook Time: 25 Minutes

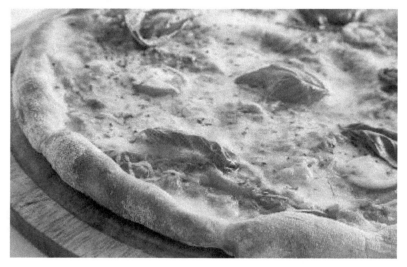

Ingredients:

For the crust, you need the following ingredients;

- 4 large eggs,
- 6 oz. of shredded (mozzarella preferred),

For the topping, you need the following ingredients;

- 3 ½ tablespoons of tomato paste,
- 1 tablespoon of dried oregano,
- 4 oz. of shredded cheese,
- 1 ¾ oz. of Pepperoni, and,
- Some olives

For the serving, you need the following ingredients;

- ½ lbs. of leafy green veggies,
- 2 tablespoons of olive oil, and
- ½ teaspoon of salt.

Directions:

Pre-heat the oven to about 400-degree F, then get a bowl and inside, beat the eggs and blend some 6 ounces of cheese. Spread the cheese and egg batter on top of a baking sheet, which has been line with a parchment paper. You should be able to form 2 rounds of pizza circles, otherwise you can just make a single rectangular pizza. Bake the pizza in the oven for about 15 minutes until it turns golden brown. Remove the pizza and let it cool down for about 10 minutes. While the pizza is cooling off, increase the oven temperature to around 450 degree F. spread the tomato crust on top of the crust, before sprinkling the oregano at the top. Top up the pizza with some 4 ounces of cheese before placing the pepperoni and olives on the top. Bake the pizza for extra 8 minutes until the pizza turns dark brown. You can serve immediately after cooling, with some salad.

Nutritional Information per Serving:

Calories: 269; Total Fat: 22 g; Carbs: 15 g; Dietary Fiber: 4 g;
Protein: 8 g; Cholesterol: 63 mg; Sodium: 147 mg

17. KETOGENIC EGG MUFFINS

Yield: 4 Servings

Total Time: 30 Minutes

Prep Time: 10 Minutes

Cook Time: 20 Minutes

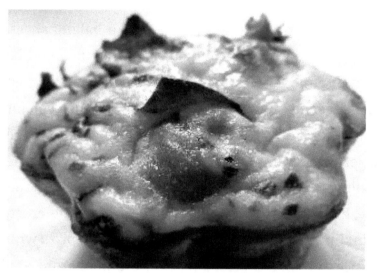

Ingredients;

- 6 large eggs,
- 2 finely chopped scallions,
- 5 thinly sliced of air-dried chorizo or bacon (cooked),
- 3 oz. of shredded cheese,
- Optional 1 ¼ tablespoons of red or green pesto,
- ½ teaspoon of salt
- ½ teaspoon of pepper

Directions:

Pre-heat the oven to about 350-degree F, then chop the scallions and bacon. Get a new bowl, and inside, whisk the eggs alongside the pesto and seasonings. Add the cheese and stir the mix very well. Simply place the batter inside the muffin cups, and add the bacon, salami or chorizo. Bake the muffin for about 20 minutes or less, depending on the size of the muffin.

Nutritional Information per Serving:

Calories: 217; Total Fat: 19 g; Carbs: 3 g; Dietary Fiber: 3 g; Protein: 7 g; Cholesterol: 0 mg; Sodium: 0 mg

18. KETOGENIC PARMESAN CROUTONS

Yield: 8 Servings

Total Time: 1 Hour

Prep Time: 15 Minutes

Cook Time: 45 Minutes

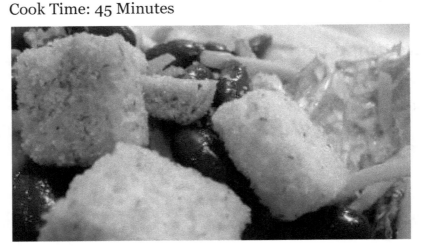

Ingredients:

- 1 ½ cups of almond flour,
- 4 ½ tablespoons of ground psyllium husk powder,
- 2 ½ teaspoons of baking powder,
- 1 teaspoon of salt,
- 2 ½ teaspoons of white wine vinegar or apple cider vinegar,
- 1 ½ cups of boiling water, and
- 3 large eggs.

For the Parmesan topping, you need the following ingredients:

- 3 oz. of butter, and
- 2 oz. of grated parmesan cheese.

Direction

Pre-heat your oven to 350 degree F. get a large bowl and inside, mix all the dry ingredients. Bring the water to a boil, and add the egg whites and vinegar, then whisk inside the bowl, with the aid of a hand mixer, for about 30 seconds (make sure the dough is not over-mixed). Form the dough into 8 pieces of flat dough with your moisty hand, and keep in mind that you need to create sufficient spaces in-between the dough, because their sizes will double after baking.

Bake the dough on the lower rack of the oven for about 40 minutes, then let them cool for few minutes before splitting the bread in equal halves. Stir the butter and parmesan cheese together, and spread on top of the bread and then raise the temperature of the oven to 450-degree F and make sure the broil function is on. Broil your bread pieces for about 5 minutes until they turn golden brown, and cool them for a while before serving it immediately as a snack or with your favorite keto salad or soup.

Nutritional Information per Serving:

Calories: 269; Total Fat: 22 g; Carbs: 15 g; Dietary Fiber: 4 g;
Protein: 8 g; Cholesterol: 63 mg; Sodium: 147 mg

19. KETOGENIC ENGLISH MUFFINS

Yield: 3 Servings

Total Time: 15 Minutes

Prep Time: 10 Minutes

Cook Time: 5 Minutes

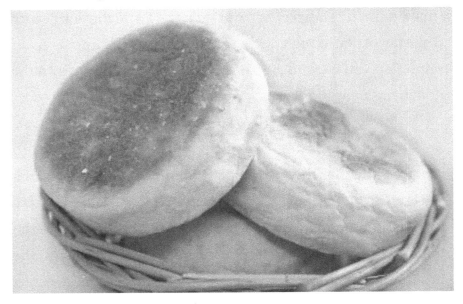

Ingredients:

- 2 eggs,
- 2 ½ tablespoons of coconut flour,
- ½ a teaspoon of baking powder,
- ½ teaspoon of salt, and
- 2 ½ tablespoons of butter or coconut oil (you need this for frying).

Directions:

Get a bowl and mix together baking powder, with salt, and coconut flour. Crack your eggs inside the bowl, and then whisk together, and let the mix sit together for few minutes. Place the three dollops of the batter you created, inside a frying pan containing butter and then heat at medium levels. Turn the bread to the other side after few minutes, and fry for few minutes. Serve the bread with butter and with your favorite topping.

This special bread can also be enjoyed with cooked beans, stew, or soup.

Nutritional Information per Serving:

Calories: 217; Total Fat: 19 g; Carbs: 3 g; Dietary Fiber: 3 g; Protein: 7 g; Cholesterol: 0 mg; Sodium: 0 mg

20. *KETOGENIC HOT DOGS*

Yield: 4 Servings

Total Time: 50 Minutes

Prep Time: 25 Minutes

Cook Time: 25 Minutes

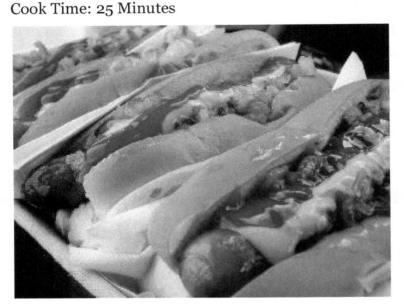

Ingredients:

- 7 ½ teaspoons of almond flour,
- 3 ½ teaspoons of coconut flour,
- ½ a teaspoon of salt,
- 1 teaspoon of baking powder,
- 2 oz. of butter,
- 2 cups of shredded cheese,
- 1 large egg,
- 8 great quality sausages (hot dog shaped),
- 1 large egg for dough brushing, and
- Optional 16 cloves of "Mummy's eyes"

Directions:

Pre-heat your oven to about 350-degree F, then get a bowl, and mix the almond flour, coconut flour, and the baking powder. Get a pan and inside, melt the butter and cheese over a low heat. Stir the cheese thoroughly when you are heating with the aid of a wooden spoon, in order to achieve a smooth batter- this should take some few minutes.

Remove the mix from the heat then crack the egg inside and stir for few seconds before adding the flour mix, then mi the whole ingredients together until they form a solid dough. Fatten the dough into a rectangle of about 8 x 14 inches. Cut the batter into 8
long strips, and make sure the strips are less than 1 inch in width. Wrap the strips of dough around the hot dogs and then brush them with whisked egg.

Line the baking sheet with parchment paper before lining the hot dogs inside, then bake for about 25 minutes until the hot dogs have turned golden brown. Add two cloves into each of the hot dogs (they will look like eyes), and make sure you don't eat those cloves, they are just for decorations.

Nutritional Information per Serving:

Calories: 269; Total Fat: 22 g; Carbs: 15 g; Dietary Fiber: 4 g;

Protein: 8 g; Cholesterol: 63 mg; Sodium: 147 mg

21. KETOGENIC BULLETPROOF BREAD RECIPE

Yield: 12 Servings

Total Time: 1 Hour

Prep Time: 20 Minutes

Cook Time: 40 Minutes

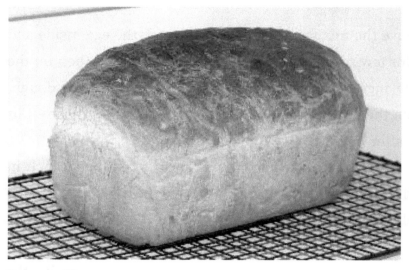

Ingredients:

- 6 separated pastured eggs,
- ½ a cup of grass-fed collagen protein, and
- Grass-fed butter.

Directions:

Pre-heat your oven to about 325-degrees, and make use of the middle rack for this baking (remove racks above the bread as the bread will expand rapidly during baking). Butter the loaf pan or dish with the butter (you may want to make use of a ceramic pan if necessary because the bread will bake evenly without any sticking problem) you need to take note also that ceramic pans will not cause the leaching of certain chemicals such as the Teflon cookware chemicals.

Get a bowl and beat the eggs until it becomes stiff, and peaks, you may also make use of a hand mixer, in place of a bowl with a spoon. Make sure the eggs are beaten perfectly, if you don't, they may collapse especially when the whey and egg yolks are added, and you will end up with a concoction that is unsightly. Add the collage protein, along the egg yolks, then blend gently on low mixing, until the mix becomes fully incorporated. The batter should become fluffy after this mixing.

Pour your batter inside the baking pan, and place in the oven. Bake the bread dough for about 40 minutes. Remove the baked bread and place on a rack to allow it cool for few minutes. As the baked bread is cooling the loaf will sink gently into the normal height after expanding rapidly under oven heat. Once the bread has cooled, simply remove it from the rack and slice before serving. You may want to keep the leftovers inside the refrigerator.

Nutritional Information per Serving:

Calories: 269; Total Fat: 22 g; Carbs: 15 g; Dietary Fiber: 4 g;

Protein: 8 g; Cholesterol: 63 mg; Sodium: 147 mg

22. *KETO WAFFLE*

Yield: 4 Servings

Total Time: 30 Minutes

Prep Time: 20 Minutes

Cook Time: 10 Minutes

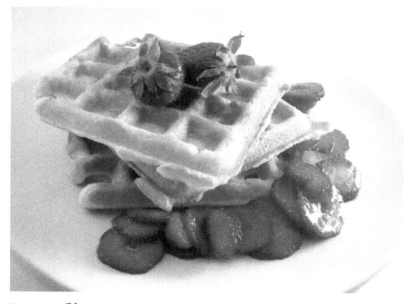

Ingredients:

- 2 large eggs,
- 2 ounces of cream cheese, or 2 tablespoons of Mayo,
- 2 tablespoons of your ketogenic toppings (sugar-free syrup or butter preferred).

Directions:

Get your blender or a magic bullet, and inside, toss the eggs alongside the cream cheese. You don't have to bring the ingredients to room temperature. Blend the cheese and egg mix until you are able to achieve a thin and bubbly batter. Allow the batter to rest for some minutes (about 5 minutes), and while this is going on, bring out your Waffle maker, and pre-heat it for about 5 minutes. When the Waffle maker is hot, and once the waffle maker has been heated up, simply pour the batch inside it (the size of the batch you pour should depend on the size of the waffle maker).

If you don't have a huge Cuisinart waffle maker, you need to adjust the pouring of the waffle batch, and sometimes you may have to make two batches of waffle (if you are making something for your friends and family). Close the waffle maker lid, and wait for a few moments until you no longer see any steam coming out. Put on the waffle plate and then top up if necessary. Serve the waffles immediately.

You need to take note of the fact that these waffles may not come out as crispy as some other waffles, however, they will come out better and crispier if you make use of a toaster oven, this simply means, you can make use of the waffle maker, and then toast them inside the toaster oven anytime you want.

Nutritional Information per Serving:

Calories: 269; Total Fat: 22 g; Carbs: 15 g; Dietary Fiber: 4 g;

Protein: 8 g; Cholesterol: 63 mg; Sodium: 147 mg

Chapter 8 - Keto

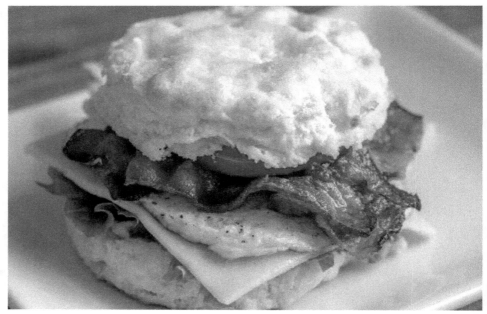

Breakfast Breads

The delicious recipes featured in this chapter would be the perfect for those of us who love breads, waffles and sandwiches but not sure how to incorporate healthier types of breads while maintaining your Ketogenic nutritional daily requirements.

Thank you for allowing us to expose you to the large variety of Keto Bread recipes that you can enjoy, please feel free to leave us a positive review if you like what you are about to read through.

23. KETOGENIC BACON EGG WITH CHEESE MUFFINS

Yield: 12 Servings

Total Time: 30 Minutes

Prep Time: 10 Minutes

Cook Time: 20 Minutes

Ingredients:

- 1 cup of cottage cheese,
- ¾ cup of grated Parmesan cheese,
- ¼ of a cup of coconut flour,
- 2/3 of a cup of almond flour,
- 1 tablespoon of baking powder,
- ½ a teaspoon of salt,
- ½ a cup of water,
- 5 beaten eggs,
- 3 stripped bacon, and
- ½ a cup of shredded cheddar cheese.

Directions:

Pre-heat your oven to about 400-degree F, and grease your muffin cups. Get a mixing bowl and inside mix the cottage cheese, with Parmesan cheese, almond flour, coconut flour, salt, water, baking powder, and the egg that has just been beaten. Mix the crumbled bacon alongside the cheddar cheese. Fill up the muffin cups until they are half or ¾ full, then sprinkle the muffin tops with extra cheddar cheese (shredded) - this is optional. Bake for about 30 minutes, until the muffins have become light brown and serve them hot or cool for few minutes at room temperature before serving.

Nutritional Information per Serving:

Calories: 217; Total Fat: 19 g; Carbs: 3 g; Dietary Fiber: 3 g; Protein: 7 g; Cholesterol: 0 mg; Sodium: 0 mg

24. SUGAR-FREE KETO BAGEL

Yield: 4-8 Servings

Total Time: 40 Minutes

Prep Time: 15 Minutes

Cook Time: 25 Minutes

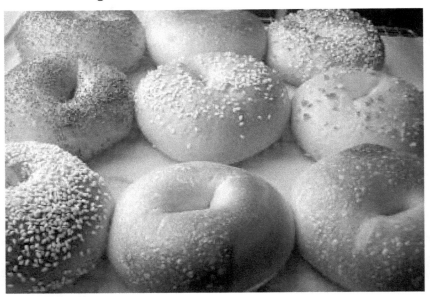

Ingredients:

- 12 medium to large eggs,
- 1/3 of a cup of sour cream,
- ¼ of a cup of ground flaxseed,
- ½ a teaspoon of sea salt,
- 1 teaspoon of baking powder,
- 1/3 of a cup of coconut flour,
- 2 scoops or 1 cup of protein powder,
- 1 teaspoon of parsley (dried),
- 1 teaspoon of Oregano (dried),
- 1 teaspoon of minced onion (dried),
- ½ a teaspoon of garlic powder

- ½ a teaspoon of dried basil, and
- ½ a teaspoon of sea salt.

Directions:

Pre-heat your oven to about 350 degrees, then get a stand mixer and inside, mix the egg and sour cream and blend perfectly until they are perfectly combined. Get a new bowl and inside, mix the flaxseed, baking powder, salt, protein powder and the coconut powder together. Pour the dry ingredients into the wet ones slowly inside the stand mixer until they are perfectly mixed. Get a small bowl, and inside, mix the ingredients for the seasoning together and set aside for few minutes. Grease a dough pan that can accommodate between 6 and 8 bagels, and sprinkle 1 teaspoon each of the seasoning unto each section of the Bagel before pouring the batter evenly unto the sections. Spread the remainder of the seasoning evenly on the bagels, and unto the batter. Bake the bagels for about 25 minutes until they begin to turn golden-brown in color. Remove the bagels from the pan and cool them or keep them in the refrigerator until you want to toast and consume them.

Nutritional Information per Serving:

Calories: 141; Total Fat: 12 g; Carbs: 2 g; Dietary Fiber: 0 g; Protein: 4 g; Cholesterol: 0 mg; Sodium: 0 mg

25. LOW CARB 5-INGREDIENT CHIP WAFFLES

Yield: 2 Servings

Total Time: 25 Minutes

Prep Time: 10 Minutes

Cook Time: 15 Minutes

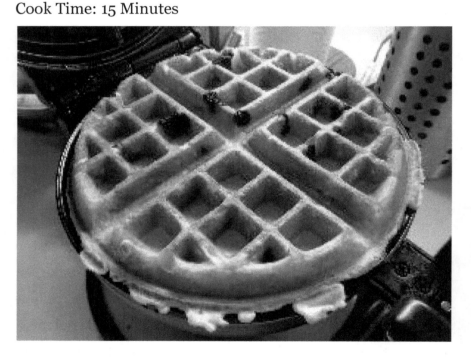

Ingredients:

- 2 scoops of vanilla pure protein powder,
- 2 separated large eggs,
- 2 melted tablespoons of butter,
- ½ teaspoon of sea salt,
- 50grams of sugar-free chocolate chips,
- ½ a cup of Walden Farm Maple syrup.

Directions:

Get a medium to large bowl and inside, whisk the egg white until it becomes stiff, then get another bowl and inside, mix the scoops of vanilla protein powder with the egg yolk, and melted butter and whisk together. You may want to thin-out the batter of necessary, by adding some water. Fold the egg whites inside the last mix, before adding the sugar-free chocolate chips and salt. Pour the waffle batter inside the waffle maker, and cook the waffle according to the instructions from the waffle maker manufacturer.

Nutritional Information per Serving:

Calories: 269; Total Fat: 22 g; Carbs: 15 g; Dietary Fiber: 4 g;
Protein: 8 g; Cholesterol: 63 mg; Sodium: 147 mg

26. KETO HAZELNUT CHOCOLATE CHIP SCONES

Yield: 12 Servings

Total Time: 1 Hour

Prep Time: 30 Minutes

Cook Time: 30 Minutes

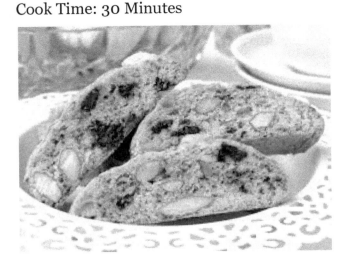

Ingredients:

- 2 ¾ cups of Hazelnut meal,
- ½ a cup of golden flax seed meal,
- 1/3 of a cup of swerve or stevia sweetener,
- 1 tablespoon of baking powder,
- 1 pinch of salt,
- 2 medium to large eggs,
- ¼ of a cup of Hazelnut oil,
- 2 tablespoons of cream,
- ½ a teaspoon of hazelnut extract (or vanilla extract),
- ¼ of a teaspoon of stevia extract, and
- 1/3 of a cup of sugar-free chocolate chips (Lily's preferred) and

- An optional 1 tablespoon of butter, with 2 oz. of dark chocolate for the chocolate drizzle.

Directions:

For the scones, simply pre-heat the oven to about 325-degree F, and then line your baking sheet with parchment paper. Get a large bowl, and inside whisk together the flax seed meal, with the hazelnut meal, sweetener, salt, and baking powder. Add the hazelnut oil, eggs, extract, and cream, then mix perfectly until the dough has formed together perfectly, then stir in your chocolate chips.

Turn the dough into the baking sheet before pat it into the rough rectangle and make it an inch thick. With the aid of a knife, simply cut the dough into 6 equal squares before cutting each square diagonally into triangles. Gently, separate and lift the scones before placing them on the baking sheet and then leave about an inch between each scone then bake for about 25 minutes until the cones are quite firm when touched and has been lightly browned. Remove the scones from the oven and let them cool for about 5 minutes.

For the chocolate drizzle, get a small pan and set it over simmering water, then melt the butter and chocolate inside the pan until the mi becomes smooth. Drizzle the mix over the scones, and let them set for about 20 minutes.

Nutritional Information per Serving:

Calories: 269; Total Fat: 22 g; Carbs: 15 g; Dietary Fiber: 4 g;

Protein: 8 g; Cholesterol: 63 mg; Sodium: 147 mg

27. THE ULTIMATE KETOGENIC BAGEL

Yield: 1 Servings

Total Time: 1 Hour 20 Minutes

Prep Time: 20 Minutes

Cook Time: 1 Hour

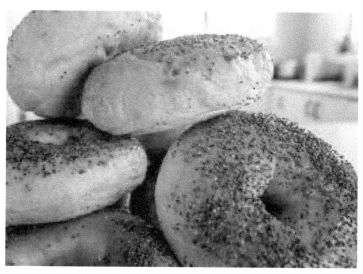

Ingredients:

- 1 ¼ cup of coconut flour,
- ¼ of a cup of Psyllium fiber,
- ½ a cup of sesame seeds,
- ½ a cup of hemp hearts,
- ½ a cup of pumpkin seeds,
- 6 eggs (organic egg whites),
- 1 teaspoon of salt, and
- 1 tablespoon of baking powder (make sure they are aluminum free).

Directions:

Pre-heat your oven to about 350-degree F, and then get a bowl where you can combine all the dry ingredients- mix the ingredients well. Get a blender, and inside gently blend the egg whites until they generate some foam (you can make use of a food processor for the same purpose. Add the foamy egg white unto the dry ingredients, then mix perfectly with the aid of a spoon, alternatively, you can make use of a food processor.

Make sure the final dough is crumbly, then add a cup of water unto the dough and continue to stir until the dough is formed- but make sure it will stick together when formed into a ball. Place a sheet of parchment paper inside the cookie sheet, then form

the dough into 6 different balls. Holding the ball in one hand gently stick your thumb through the center for create a hole before placing the dough inside the cookie sheet in order to form a bagel. Make sure you press the dough together with your fingers.

Sprinkle some sesame seeds on top of the bagel, to make it look even more fascinating. Bake the bagel at about 350 degree for about 55 minutes, and let it cool inside the oven after baking, in order to create a crunchy top. Serve the bagels immediately.

Nutritional Information per Serving:

Calories: 141; Total Fat: 12 g; Carbs: 2 g; Dietary Fiber: 0 g; Protein: 4 g; Cholesterol: 0 mg; Sodium: 0 mg

28. KETOGENIC HAM & CHEESE STUFFED WAFFLE

Yield: 4 Servings

Total Time: 30 Minutes

Prep Time: 20 Minutes

Cook Time: 10 Minutes

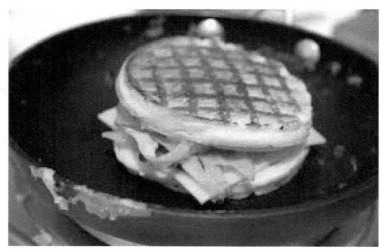

Ingredients;

- 6 tablespoons of unsweetened coconut or almond milk,
- ½ a teaspoon of apple cider vinegar,
- 2 medium or large eggs,
- 1 tablespoon of coconut or olive oil, ½ teaspoon of vanilla GF extract,
- ¾ of a cup of almond flour,
- 2 tablespoons of coconut flour,
- 2 teaspoons of corn-free baking powder,
- 2 teaspoon of natural low carb sweetener (erythritol or coconut sugar are mostly prepared),
- 4 slices of deli ham, and
- 4 slice of cheddar cheese.

Directions:

Pre-heat tor waffle maker to medium-high after oiling it, unless you come with a non-sticky waffle maker. Get a large bowl and inside mix the coconut or almond milk with the apple cider vinegar, mi very well and add the mix to a mixture of egg, coconut or olive oil and vanilla extract, then mix thoroughly before setting it aside. Get a second large bowl and inside add the almond flour with the coconut flour baking powder and sweetener and whisk everything together.

Add your dry flour mix to the wet and whisk thoroughly together. Pour a quarter of the waffle into the waffle maker, and with the aid of a spoon, spread the batter evenly and then place 2 slices of ham on top as well as 2 slices of cheese over the batter, and then add a little more batter over the top before spreading the batter to ensure that the cheese and ham are perfectly covered. Close the waffle maker and cook for about 5 minutes until steam is no longer rising from the waffle maker. Remove the waffles from the waffle maker and serve immediately.

Nutritional Information per Serving:

Calories: 181; Total Fat: 12 g; Carbs: 5 g; Dietary Fiber: 2 g; Protein: 10 g; Cholesterol: 58 mg; Sodium: 47 mg

29. KETOGENIC CHEESE AND BACON ROLLS

Yield: 6 Servings

Total Time: 30 Minutes

Prep Time: 10 Minutes

Cook Time: 20 Minutes

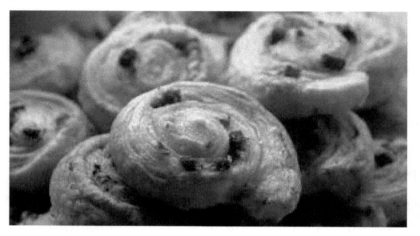

Ingredients:

- 5 ounces of Bacon (must be diced into 6),
- 2 tablespoons of cream cheese,
- 2 teaspoons of sesame seeds,
- 1 tablespoon of Psyllium seeds,
- 1 ½ teaspoons of baking powder,
- 1 cup of grated cheddar cheese,
- ½ a cup of mozzarella grated cheese,
- 3 large eggs,
- ½ teaspoon of red pepper, and
- ½ teaspoon of salt.

Directions:

Pre-heat your oven to about 355-degree F, and inside a non-sticky frying pan, sauté the diced bacon over medium heat, and until the bacon start to brown- turn off the heat at this point. Add your cream cheese inside the bacon, and allow the cheese to become soften while the bacon is cooling. Place the cream cheese alongside the bacon inside a food processor, and add the remainder of the ingredients (keep a spoonful of the bacon aside as top up for the rolls). Blend the mix in the processor at medium speed for around 5 minutes, until the ingredients become well combined. Spoon the blended mi into 12 equal piles, on a lined baking dish, before you sprinkle the reserved bacon on top of each roll. Bake the rolls for about 16 minutes, until they become puffed up and golden in color. You can store them while hot or keep them in the refrigerator and they can be quickly warmed inside the oven anytime needed.

Nutritional Information per Serving:

Calories: 81; Total Fat: 6 g; Carbs: 5 g; Dietary Fiber: 2 g; Protein: 5 g; Cholesterol: 58 mg; Sodium: 476 mg

30. COCONUT MACADAMIA BARS

Yield: 5 Servings

Total Time: 45 Minutes

Prep Time: 30 Minutes

Cook Time: 15 Minutes

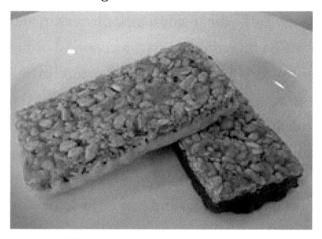

Ingredients:

- 2 cups or 60 grams of Macadamia nuts,
- ½ a cup of almond butter,
- ¼ of a cup of a cup of coconut oil,
- 5 tablespoons of shredded unsweetened coconut, and
- 15 drops of sweet leaf stevia.

Direction

Get a food processor or with the aid of your hand, simply crush the macadamia nuts. Get a mixing bowl, and inside combine the almond butter with the coconut oil, and shredded coconut. Add the stevia drops as well as the crushed macadamia nuts.

Mix the batter very well before pouring it inside a baking dish that has been lined with a parchment paper. Bake for about 15 minutes, then cool and serve immediately, otherwise you can store inside the refrigerator.

Nutritional Information per Serving:

Calories: 269; Total Fat: 22 g; Carbs: 15 g; Dietary Fiber: 4 g;

Protein: 8 g; Cholesterol: 63 mg; Sodium: 147 mg

31. KETOGENIC AVOCADO BREAKFAST PIZZA

Yield: 8 Servings

Total Time: 40 Minutes

Prep Time: 20 Minutes

Cook Time: 20 Minutes

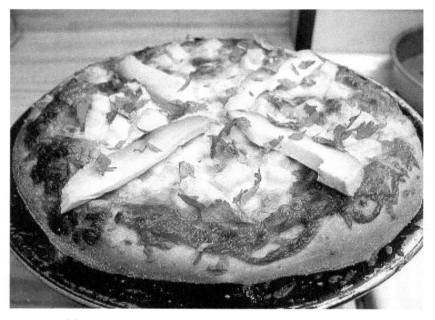

Ingredients:

- 4 large eggs,
- 1 cup of almond milk or flour,
- 1 ½ cups of shredded mozzarella cheese,
- 4 oz. of cream cheese,
- 2 large Hass avocados,
- ¼ of a cup of extra virgin olive oil,
- 4 slices of thick bacon,

- ½ a cup of shredded cheddar jack cheese,
- 1 tablespoon of unsalted butter,
- ½ a tablespoon of Italian season, and
- ½ teaspoon each of salt and pepper.

Directions:

Pre-heat your oven to about 425-degree F, then soften the cream cheese alongside the mozzarella cheese, inside the microwave for around 45 seconds, until the cheese mix are slightly melted. Add your almond flour, Italia seasoning, egg, pepper, and salt, and stir the mix until it forms a dough. Line the baking sheet with parchment paper, and before coating with a non-sticky spray. Pour the dough inside the baking sheet and with the aid of a spatula, spread the dough to form a long rectangular shape.

Bake the dough for about 12 minutes until it becomes golden light brown. Cook the bacon inside a microwave for about 5 minutes until it becomes crispy, then set aside for it to cool. Split your avocados into half, and then remove the pits before scoring the flesh with a knife.

With the aid of a spoon, gently scoop out the meat inside a food processor. Add the salt, olive oil, and pepper to the avocado meat and blend until the mix becomes smooth. Spread your avocado mix on top of the pizza crust, and before crumbling the bacon on top and then sprinkle your shredded cheese on top and return the pizza unto the oven where you will bake it for 7 more minutes until the cheese has completely melted.

Melt butter inside a separate pan over medium heat, and then fry your eggs for about 2 1/2 minutes on both sides, then add the fried eggs over the pizza before serving.

Nutritional Information per Serving:

Calories: 257; Total Fat: 25 g; Carbs: 8 g; Dietary Fiber: 4 g;

Protein: 16 g; Cholesterol: 50 mg; Sodium: 1.1 mg

32. KETO LEMON POPPY SEED PROTEIN MUFFINS

Yield: 3-4 Servings

Total Time: 1 Hour

Prep Time: 35 Minutes

Cook Time: 25 Minutes

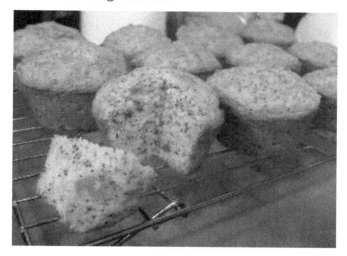

Ingredients:

- ½ a cup plus 2 tablespoons of coconut flour,
- 1 teaspoon of Xanthan gum,
- ¾ teaspoon of baking powder,
- ¾ teaspoon of baking soda,
- ¼ teaspoon of salt,
- 1 tablespoon of poppy seed,
- 1 tablespoon of lemon zest,
- 1 tablespoon of coconut oil, or melted unsalted butter,
- 1 large egg stored at room temperature,
- 1 teaspoon of vanilla extract,

- ¼ of a cup of plain and non-fat Greek yoghurt,
- ¼ cup of agave,
- 2 tablespoons of freshly squeezed juice of lemon,
- ½ a cup of unsweetened vanilla almond milk, and
- 2 scoops of low carb protein powder (the Jamie Eason lean body protein powder is preferred).

Directions:

Pre-heat your oven to about 350 degree F, and then coat lightly, 8 muffin cups (standard sizes), with a non-sticky cooking spray. Get a medium to large bowl, and inside whisk together, the coconut flour, alongside Xanthan gum, baking powder, salt, baking soda, poppy seeds, and lemon zest, and stir properly to ensure adequate mixing.

Get a separate bowl and inside whisk together the coconut oil or butter with the vanilla, before stirring in the yoghurt until there are no large lumps remaining. Stir inside the agave, alongside the almond milk, and lemon juice, then mix the protein powder into the mix. Add the coconut flour mix, then stir the entire mix until they are perfectly blended. Let the batter sit for about 10 minutes. Divide your batter in-between your prepared muffin cups, and then bake them for about 24 minutes inside the 350 degree F oven, and insert a toothpick after baking, if it comes out clean then the muffins are done. Cool the muffins inside a pan for about 5 minutes before you turn them out into the wire rack.

Nutritional Information per Serving:

Calories: 217; Total Fat: 19 g; Carbs: 3 g; Dietary Fiber: 3 g; Protein: 7 g; Cholesterol: 0 mg; Sodium: 0 mg

33. GLUTEN-FREE LOW-CARB CINNAMON FAUX-ST CRUNCH CEREAL

Yield: 6 Servings

Total Time: 2 Hours

Prep Time: 45 Minutes

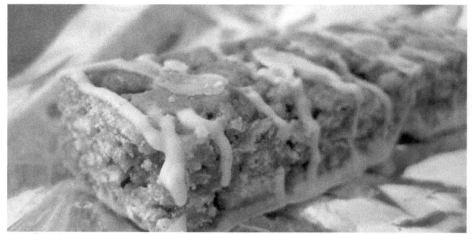

Cook Time: 1 Hour 15 Minutes

Ingredients:

- ½ a cup of flax seed (milled),
- ½ a cup of hemp seeds (hulled),
- 2 tablespoons of ground cinnamon,
- ½ a cup of apple juice, and
- 1 tablespoon of coconut oil.

Directions:

Get a blender, magic bullet or food processor, then combine all the dry ingredient inside, then add the apple juice with the coconut oil and blend perfectly well until it has achieved a smooth consistency. Put a parchment paper on cookie sheet and spread the batter on top press them down and make then thin in sizes.

Bake the batter in an oven that has been pre-heated to around 350-degree F, and for about 15 minutes. Reduce the heat to around 250-degree F and bake further for about 10 minutes.

With the aid of a knife or cutter for pizza, gently remove the baked crunch cereal from the oven and cut them into squares. Turn on the oven back and put the crunch cereal back and bake further for about an hour until they become crispy and break easily(if they remain soft after baking for about an hour, simply return to the oven and bake until it is completely crispy and dried. You may want to serve them with unsweetened almond or coconut milk.

Nutritional Information per Serving:

Calories: 269; Total Fat: 22 g; Carbs: 15 g; Dietary Fiber: 4 g;
Protein: 8 g; Cholesterol: 63 mg; Sodium: 147 mg

34. KETOGENIC CHOCOLATE-HAZELNUT PROTEIN WAFFLES

Yield: 6-10 Servings

Total Time: 1 Hour

Prep Time: 45 Minutes

Cook Time: 15 Minutes

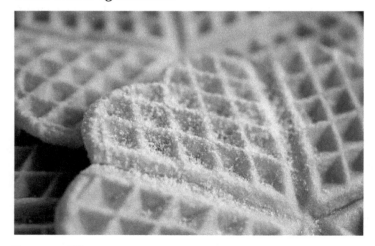

Ingredients:

- 1 ¼ cups of Hazelnut meal,
- ½ a cup of chocolate protein powder,
- 2 tablespoons of cocoa powder,
- 2 tablespoons of coconut flour,
- 3 tablespoons of swerve natural sweetener (a granulated erythritol),
- 4 eggs,
- 1/3 of a cup of Greek yoghurt (Full fat),
- 2 2/3 tablespoons of hazelnut oil ,
- ½ teaspoon of hazelnut extract, and
- ¼ tablespoon of extract of stevia.

Directions:

Pre-heat the waffle iron to meat, and then pre-heat the oven to about 200-degree F. place a wire rack on top of the baking sheet. Gt a large bowl, and inside, whisk together the protein powder, alongside the hazelnut meal, sweetener, coconut flour and the cocoa powder. Get another small to medium bowl and inside, whisk the egg alongside the yoghurt, hazelnut oil, stevia and hazelnut extract and mix perfectly well until they are properly combined.

If necessary you can grease the waffle iron and then pour a quarter of the batter into each section of the waffle iron, close the waffle iron and then cook the waffles until they become light brown and crispy in texture. Gently transfer the cooked waffles unto the baking sheet in the oven in order to keep them warm. Cook the remaining batter inside the waffle iron and then transfer them into the oven. Top up the waffles with butter, berries, whipped cream, sugar-free syrup, and serve.

Nutritional Information per Serving:

Calories: 81; Total Fat: 6 g; Carbs: 5 g; Dietary Fiber: 2 g; Protein: 5 g; Cholesterol: 58 mg; Sodium: 476 mg

35. KETOGENIC CAULIFLOWER HASH BROWNS

Yield: 4 Servings

Total Time: 20 Minutes

Prep Time: 10 Minutes

Cook Time: 10 Minutes

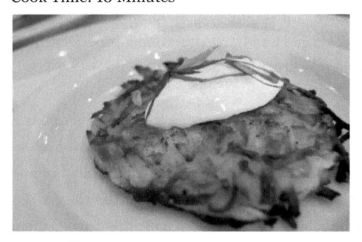

Ingredients:

- 2 cups of steamed and grated cups of cauliflower,
- ½ large chopped sweet onion,
- ¼ of a cup of parmesan cheese,
- 1 large egg,
- 3 ½ tablespoons of olive oil (divided), and
- ¼ teaspoon of salt.

Directions:

Get a 10-inch non-stick skillet, then heat a tablespoon of the olive oil inside, before sautéing the chopped onion until they turn lightly golden in color. Measure the 2 cups of the cauliflower that has been steamed, inside a colander or inside a sieve and gently press until the excess moisture has been removed completely. Gently place your cauliflower inside a medium mixing bowl, then add the Parmesan alongside the onion, into the cauliflower and stir together, then stir in the eggs and mix the entire mixture until it becomes very thick.

Warm the remaining 2 tablespoons of olive oil inside the pan and then add the cauliflower mix before cooking over medium heat for about 5 minutes until the hash browns become caramelized at the bottom- turn them over gently and make them brown by cooking for 4 minutes.

Nutritional Information per Serving:

Calories: 81; Total Fat: 6 g; Carbs: 5 g; Dietary Fiber: 2 g; Protein: 5 g; Cholesterol: 58 mg; Sodium: 476 mg

36. KETOGENIC MORNING BAR

Yield: 4-6 Servings

Total Time: 40 Minutes

Prep Time: 20 Minutes

Cook Time: 20 Minutes

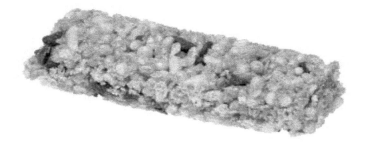

Ingredients:

- 2 ½ cups of mixed nuts and seeds (you can combine walnuts, sunflower seeds, almonds and hazelnuts, with macadamia nuts),
- ½ a cup of flaxseeds,
- 2 tablespoons of almond butter ,
- 2 large eggs,
- 1 tablespoon of Truvia natural sweetener,
- 1 tablespoon of zero sugar vanilla extract,
- An optional pinch of Cinnamon or pumpkin pie spice.

Directions:

Pre-heat the oven to about 350-degree F, and blitz your mixture of nuts and seeds inside a blender or with the aid of a hand-held beater- make sure you don't pulverize the mix and the reason being that you want the final texture to appear crunchy, therefore you need to keep some big bits mixed with the smaller ones. Add the remaining ingredients and give a thorough mixing in order to achieve a denser and sticky mixture.

Get a small baking tray and line it with a parchment paper, then pour the mix inside the baking tray and press gently down before distributing the mix evenly in a single dense layer, inside the baking tray. Bake the mix for about 20 minutes until it turns into a golden brown. With the aid of a sharp knife, cut the baked mix into 16 pieces or bars and cool them before serving, or prepare the chocolate drizzle first.

Nutritional Information per Serving:

Calories: 269; Total Fat: 22 g; Carbs: 15 g; Dietary Fiber: 4 g;
Protein: 8 g; Cholesterol: 63 mg; Sodium: 147 mg

37. KETOGENIC PUMPKIN BAGELS

Yield: 8 Servings

Total Time: 35 Minutes

Prep Time: 10 Minutes

Cook Time: 25 Minutes

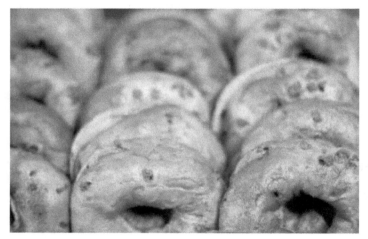

Ingredients:

- 1/3 of a cup of coconut flour (sifted),
- 3 tablespoons of golden flax meal,
- 3 beaten eggs,
- 2 tablespoons of butter (or melted coconut oil),
- ¼ of a cup of unsweetened coconut or almond milk,
- ½ a cup of pumpkin puree ,
- ¾ teaspoon of vanilla extract (organic and gluten free),
- 1 teaspoon of pumpkin pie spice,
- ½ a teaspoon of Cinnamon,
- ¼ of a teaspoon of sea salt,

- ½ of a tablespoon of sweetener (this could be honey or maple syrup),
- ½ teaspoon of baking soda(mix this with ½ teaspoon of apple cider vinegar, inside a separate bowl),
- Some kitchen tools, including bagel/donut pan,

Direction

Pre-heat the oven to about 350 degree F and then oil or grease the bagel or donut pan. Get a large mixing bowl, and inside, combine the golden flax meal with the sifted coconut flour, pumpkin pie spice, cinnamon, and the sea salt, then mix all the ingredients very well. Get a separate mixing bowl, and inside, mix the pumpkin puree with the eggs, milk, sweetener, vanilla extract, and melted butter or coconut oil.

In a separate bowl, mix the apple cider vinegar with the baking soda and then add the egg mixture, and stir the entire mix thoroughly until a smoot batter is formed. Spoon the batter into the pan and then spread it with the back of the spoon or a spatula, then place in the oven and bake for about 25 minutes until the top of the bagel become brown and firm. Remove the pan from the oven and cool until you can remove it completely from the pan. With the aid of a butter knife simply separate the bagel from the pan edges and slide it around until you are able to lift the bagel completely out.

You can serve the bagel whole or slice into half but make sure you don't apply too much pressure. You may want to refrigerate the bagel overnight to create a firmer texture. For the perfect low carb meal, you can serve the bagel with a rub of butter or some cream cheese.

Nutritional Information per Serving:

Calories: 141; Total Fat: 12 g; Carbs: 2 g; Dietary Fiber: 0 g; Protein: 4 g; Cholesterol: 0 mg; Sodium: 0 mg

38. KETOGENIC PEANUT BUTTER BREAKFAST BARS

Yield: 12 Servings

Total Time: 1 Hour

Prep Time: 40 Minutes

Cook Time: 20 Minutes

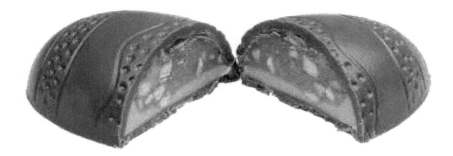

Ingredients:

- 1 cup of chunky peanut butter,
- ½ a cup of sweetener,
- ½ a cup of flax seed meal,
- ½ a cup of almond meal,
- ½ a cup of chocolate chips (zero sugar),
- 2 large egg whites,
- ½ a cup of cashews,
- ½ cup of almonds,
- ½ a teaspoon of chia seeds.

Directions:

Pre-heat the oven to about 350-degree F then line an 8 x 8 pan or a baking dish with a parchment paper make sure you leave an extra space on the sides that you can use as handles when removing the bars after baking. Get a large bowl, then mix all the ingredients until they are perfectly combined. Pour the batter inside the 8 x 8 pan and press it down into the pan so that it becomes flattened. Bake the batter for about 15 minutes Let the baked bars cool for about 5 minutes before refrigerating for about 30 minutes, then cut into bars serve all or keep the remaining bars inside the refrigerator until needed.

Nutritional Information per Serving:

Calories: 269; Total Fat: 22 g; Carbs: 15 g; Dietary Fiber: 4 g;
Protein: 8 g; Cholesterol: 63 mg; Sodium: 147 mg

39. KETO EASY ZUCCHINI FRITTERS

Yield: 8 Servings

Total Time: 30 Minutes

Prep Time: 20 Minutes

Cook Time: 10 Minutes

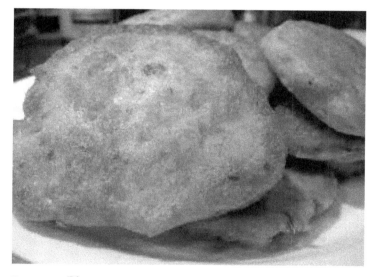

Ingredients

- 1 lb. of Zucchini (an equivalent size of summer squash can also be used),
- ¾ of a teaspoon of salt,
- 2 medium or large eggs,
- 1 ½ oz. of onion or 2 medium minced scallions,
- 1 teaspoon of lemon pepper,
- ¾ of a teaspoon of baking powder,
- ½ a cup of almond flour (Honeyville brand preferred),
- ¼ of a cup of oat fiber,

- ¼ of a cup of parmesan cheese (grated), and
- 2 tablespoons of oil for frying.

Directions:

Grate the zucchini inside the box grater or inside a food processor, then put it inside a colander before sprinkling it with the salt. Mix the zucchini very well in order to distribute the salt properly before settling it down for about 5 minutes.

Gently squeeze the zucchini properly with your hands, before placing it inside a medium-size mixing bowl. Add the scallions and eggs into the zucchini before mixing properly, then get a small bowl and inside, add all the dry ingredients and mix thoroughly.

Stir the dry ingredients together before adding the mix to the zucchini, then mix the whole thing thoroughly. Get a large pan and heat it over medium heat, then add sufficient oil to cover the bottom of the pan completely, before you increase the heat to high. Simply stick the end of a wooden spoon inside the oil just to check for bubbles, then if you discover the bubbles are moving speedily, then the oil should be hot enough.

Stir in your zucchini mix, before dipping a ¼ measuring cup inside the batter. Gently dump the batter inside the frying pan and then push it into shape, with a spatula or flipper before you cook further for about 3 minutes, while flipping up and down and then cook further for about 3 minutes.

You may add more oil if you feel you need to avoid sticking. Once cooked, drain the zucchini fritters on a paper towel before you serve.

Nutritional Information per Serving:

Calories: 81; Total Fat: 6 g; Carbs: 5 g; Dietary Fiber: 2 g; Protein: 5 g; Cholesterol: 58 mg; Sodium: 476 mg

40. LOW CARB CREAM CHEESE, HAM AND DILL PICKLE ROLLS

Yield: 2 Servings

Total Time: 5 Minutes

Prep Time: 5 Minutes

Cook Time: 0 Minutes

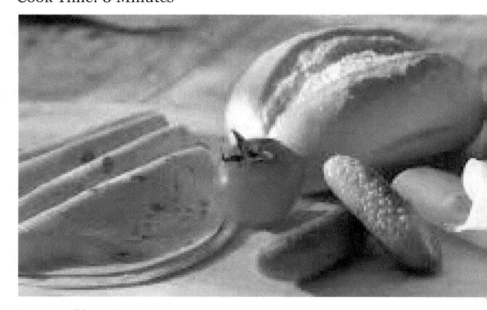

Ingredients:

- 2 oz. cooked boneless fresh ham,
- 2 tablespoons of cream cheese,
- 2 spears pickles.

Direction

Spread the cream cheese on the slices of ham, then place the pickle spear at one part or end of the slice of ham and roll up immediately. You may want to secure the rolls with tooth pick if you desire. Serve the rolls immediately and enjoy.

Nutritional Information per Serving:

Calories: 269; Total Fat: 22 g; Carbs: 15 g; Dietary Fiber: 4 g;

Protein: 8 g; Cholesterol: 63 mg; Sodium: 147 mg

41. LOW CARB WRAPPED MINI MEATLOAVES

Yield: 4 Servings

Total Time: 40 Minutes

Prep Time: 10 Minutes

Cook Time: 30 Minutes

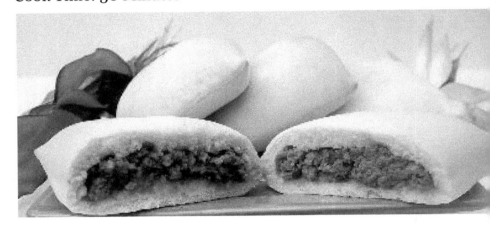

Ingredients:

- 1 lb. of 85% lean ground beef,
- ¾ of a teaspoon of kosher salt,
- ¼ of a teaspoon of black pepper,
- 1 teaspoon of garlic powder,
- 1 teaspoon of onion powder,
- 1 teaspoon of smoked paprika,
- 1 teaspoon of chili powder,
- 1 teaspoon of parsley (dried),
- 8 bacon strips (thin)

Directions:

Pre-heat the oven to about 400-degree F, and get a medium bowl and inside mix together the ground beef with the spices. Divide the mix into 8 different but equal parts. Line some 8 muffin cups with the bacon, in such a way that each cup will be circled by the strip of the bacon, then place each of the mini meatloaf inside the circle of within the strips of bacon. Bake them for about 30 minutes and when done, simply transfer the cooked meatloaf unto some paper towels to drain before serving.

Nutritional Information per Serving:

Calories: 269; Total Fat: 22 g; Carbs: 15 g; Dietary Fiber: 4 g;

Protein: 8 g; Cholesterol: 63 mg; Sodium: 147 mg

42. HAM AND CHEESE CAULIFLOWER FRITTERS RECIPE

Yield: 2 Servings

Total Time: 30 Minutes

Prep Time: 20 Minutes

Cook Time: 10 Minutes

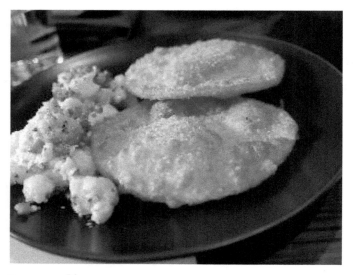

Ingredients:

- 1 medium to large cauliflower head,
- 3 eggs,
- 2 ¼ cups of grated cheddar cheese,
- 1 1/4 cups of diced ham,
- 2 ½ tablespoons of coconut flour,
- 1 clove minced garlic,
- 1 teaspoon of mustard powder,
- ½ a teaspoon of salt,

- ½ a teaspoon of pepper, and
- 2 tablespoons of oil or butter for the baking pan.

Directions:

Chop your cauliflower into pieces (½ inch each), then steam the mix for about 15 minutes, until it becomes soft. Drain the cauliflower in a fine mesh sieve then marsh it up with a fork or a potato masher, make sure you press down in order to extract as much water from the cauliflower as you can, however you must make it slightly chunky and not too smooth.

Transfer the cauliflower into a large bowl, then add the cheese, eggs, ham, garlic, coconut flour, salt, mustard, and pepper. Stir the mix perfectly well in order to create a consistent mix.

Get a large non-skillet and heat it over medium heat and then add the butter or oil inside the pan. With the use of 2 or 3 spoons at a time, gently form the cauliflower into some fat patties, and press them together in a firm manner, but make sure they don't extend beyond 3 inches in diameter measurement.

When the baking pan is hot, simply add few cauliflower patties at a time and make sure you don't get them crowded into the pan, then cook them for about 5 minutes before you remove them and place them on paper towel lined plates. Repeat the cooking for the remaining patties until they are all done. Serve the patties while they are still hot.

Nutritional Information per Serving:

Calories: 81; Total Fat: 6 g; Carbs: 5 g; Dietary Fiber: 2 g; Protein: 5 g; Cholesterol: 58 mg; Sodium: 476 mg

43. LOW CARB FISHING FRITTATAS

Yield: 6 Servings

Total Time: 20 Minutes

Prep Time: 10 Minutes

Cook Time: 10 Minutes

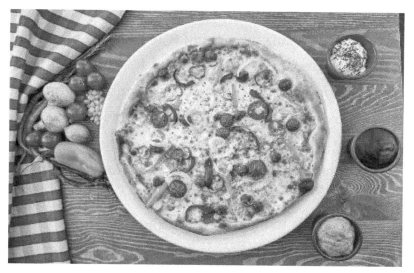

Ingredients:

- 1 tin or 3 oz. of Tuna inside olive oil,
- 1 large or 7 oz. of grated courgetti,
- 2 medium or large eggs,
- 1 tablespoon of coconut oil,
- 2 teaspoons of dried chili flakes or 1 finely chopped and fried chili,
- ½ teaspoon each of salt and pepper,
- 1/8 teaspoon of Xanthan or guar gum (this is optional).

Direction:

Simply open the tuna tin, however make sure you don't drain, but flake the tuna into smaller bits. Grate the zucchini then squeeze the excess moisture out. Add the eggs, tuna and zucchini together and then mix perfectly well. Get a bowl and inside, combine the coconut flour with the spices and the dry ingredients, before adding it into the tuna. If you are using fresh chilies, you need to chop them finely before frying them for about 2 minutes. mix everything together with the chilies and let the mix stand for about 5 minutes, take note of the fact that the addition of coconut flour to the mix will make it absorb moisture and allow the batter to become stickier.

Get a small fry pan and heat a little oil inside, and with the aid of a large spoon, add the batter into the into the pan (the batter should be able to make 6 frittatas), make sure they are at least 5mm in thickness, but if they are thicker than 5mm then you have to cook them for more time. Make sure you fry over medium to high heat for about 7 minutes. Make sure that the frittatas are lightly brown before you take them from the frying pan, and serve.

Nutritional Information per Serving:

Calories: 661; Total Fat: 59 g; Carbs: 4 g; Dietary Fiber: 1 g; Protein: 27 g; Cholesterol: 0 mg; Sodium: 0 mg

44. OMM LOW CARB FRENCH TOAST

Yield: 4 Servings

Total Time: 40 Minutes

Prep Time: 25 Minutes

Cook Time: 15 Minutes

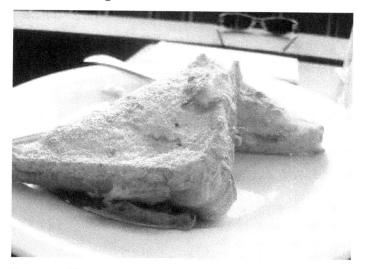

Ingredients;

- 2/3 of a cup of coconut flour,
- 1 tablespoon of natural sugar alternative such as Swerve,
- 2 teaspoons of baking powder,
- 1 teaspoon of a dash of salt,
- 8 large divided whole eggs,
- ¾ of a cup of unsweetened and divided almond milk,
- 1 teaspoon of vanilla extract,
- ¼ of a cup of melted butter,
- ½ a cup of heavy cream whipping, and

- 1/4 of a cup of fresh butter.

Directions:

Get a large bowl, and inside, mix the coconut flour with the natural sweetener, baking powder plus salt and stir very well before setting aside. Get another bowl and inside whisk together four of the eight eggs, then add just ¼ of the almond milk and the vanilla, then whisk perfectly. Add the dry ingredients to the wet ones and whisk again, while you are pouring the melted butter.

Get 12 microwaveable containers (make sure they are fairly wide), and grease them- the 8 oz. ramekins are highly recommended however, you may also make use of the flat-bottom soup bowls, or the wide coffee mugs, but you will have to cut the muffins into halves if you are using the tall coffee cups.

Pour the batter into the containers and then microwave the muffins. Take note, you should add 1 minute to the microwave for each muffin, and you can microwave in two batches (6 muffins a cup). Each batch of muffins should be in the oven for about 6 minutes, hence 12 minutes total for all the muffins. While the muffins are in the making, get another bowl and inside whisk together the remaining eggs, with the remaining almond milk, and heavy cream. As you remove the muffins from the microwave, simply pop them out and allow them to cool down for about 1 minute before (make sure they don't cook the egg mix), once they have cooled for 60 seconds, add the muffins to the egg mix and let them sit in for about few minutes and flip them occasionally. They should be fragile but still good enough to be flip around until they absorb the egg mix.

Once they are absorbing the egg mix, simply get a large skillet or a sauté pan, and place it over medium heat before adding some butter and melt. Fry the muffins inside the melted butter just like you will fry the French toast, then keep the French toast inside the oven until they are ready to be served, or simply serve hot after frying.

Nutritional Information per Serving:

Calories: 217; Total Fat: 19 g; Carbs: 3 g; Dietary Fiber: 3 g; Protein: 7 g; Cholesterol: 0 mg; Sodium: 0 mg

45. KETOGENIC PALEO EGG MCMUFFIN

Yield: 1 Servings

Total Time: 45 Minutes

Prep Time: 30 Minutes

Cook Time: 15 Minutes

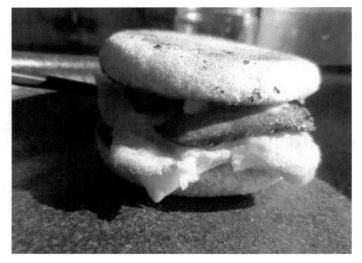

Ingredients:

- 2 tablespoons of ghee (must be divided),
- ¼ of a pound of raw pork (breakfast sausage),
- 2 medium to large eggs,
- ¼ teaspoon of salt,
- ¼ of a teaspoon of ground pepper,
- ¼ of a cup of water,
- Optional 1 heaping tablespoon of guacamole.

Directions:

Get two 3 ½ inch of stainless biscuit cutters and then grease the inside with meted ghee. Place a cutter on the plate before filling it with sausage meat. If a bulk sausage is not available you may want to cook some bacon, and make sure your press down the meat in a uniform manner, in order to shape the sausage perfectly.

Get a skillet, and then heat it over a medium before adding a tablespoon of ghee into it. Once the fat is shimmering, you can add your patty inside the pan and if you want this patty to retain its round shape, make sure you keep the mold on until the patty has cooked and shrink away by the sides. Once cook, simply lift it off and away.

Clean your biscuit cutter and then grease again before frying the sausage for about 3 minutes on each side until the mix has cooked properly. In case the patty is thick, you may want to cover the pan just to make sure the patty is fully cooked. Transfer the patty into a plate once the cooking is completed.

Now it's time to prepare the buns. To do this simply get 2 small bowls and then crack an egg into each then pierce through the yolk with the aid of a fork. Get a skillet and heat it over medium heat with the remaining ghee, and ensure that you have a tight lid on top of the fillet. Once the ghee is shimmering, simply place your 2 greased biscuit cutters inside the pan before pouring an egg into each mold. Season each egg with pepper and salt for added taste, before adding the water unto the skillet (water should be poured at the side of the egg mold and ensure that it does not enter the egg). Turn the heat down and cover.

Allow the eggs to cook for about 3 minutes before transferring them into a paper-towel lined plate. You may want to take an easier way by sliding a spatula under the mold of eggs, and tilt them up gently (make sure you wear a glove when doing this). Finally prepare the McMuffin by gently sandwiching the sausage patty in-between the egg rounds, and you can serve immediately, as a scrumptious lunch or dinner snack.

Nutritional Information per Serving:

Calories: 626; Total Fat: 54.6 g; Carbs: 2.9 g; Dietary Fiber: 6.5 g;
Protein: 26.5 g; Cholesterol: 0 mg; Sodium: 0 mg

46. KETO FLOURLESS EGG WITH COTTAGE CHEESE MUFFIN-FOR BREAKFAST

Yield: 12 Servings

Total Time: 50 Minutes

Prep Time: 20 Minutes

Cook Time: 30 Minutes

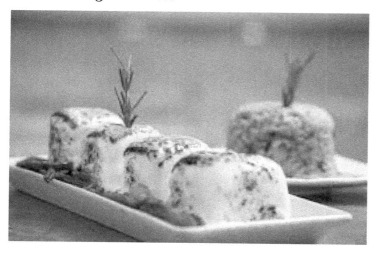

Ingredients:

- ½ a cup of almond meal (almond flour may also work but almond meal provides a coarser texture that is more desirable).
- ½ a cup of raw hemp seed,
- ½ a cup of Parmesan cheese (finely grated),
- ¼ of a cup of flax seed meal,
- ¼ of a cup of nutritional yeast flakes,
- ½ a teaspoon of baking powder,
- ½ a teaspoon of spike seasoning (this is optional but can be an ideal substitute for all-purpose seasoning), and

- ¼ of a teaspoon of salt.

The wet ingredients you will need for this recipe include;

- 6 large beaten eggs,
- ½ a cup of reduced-fat cottage cheese,
- 1/3 of a cup of thinly sliced green onion

Directions:

Pre-heat your oven to about 375 degree F and spray the muffin pans with a non-sticky spray or olive oil. If you use muffin cups larger than 2-inches in width then you may get lesser amount of muffin servings.

Get a medium sized bowl and inside, mix the almond meal with the raw hemp seed, parmesan cheese, salt, spike seasoning. Get a smaller bowl, and inside beat the eggs and mix it with the reduced-fat cottage cheese and the green onions. Mix both the wet and dry ingredients together and scoop the mix inside a measuring cup before filling up the muffin cups until they are almost filled up (make sure the scoop is evenly distributed among the muffin cups).

Bake the muffins for about 30 minutes until they are brown and firm. You may want to serve these muffins immediately or refrigerate them as they can store very well for about a week, and then re-heat them inside the microwave or toaster.

Nutritional Information per Serving:

Calories: 217; Total Fat: 19 g; Carbs: 3 g; Dietary Fiber: 3 g; Protein: 7 g; Cholesterol: 0 mg; Sodium: 0 mg

Chapter 9 – Sweet Keto Breakfast Breads

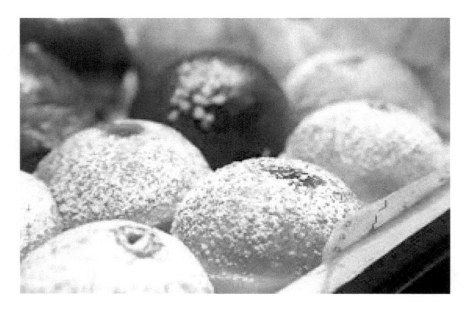

The delicious recipes featured in this chapter would be the perfect for those of us who love sweets, breads, and desserts but not sure how to incorporate healthier types of breads while maintaining your Ketogenic nutritional daily requirements.

Thank you for allowing us to expose you to the large variety of Keto Bread recipes that you can enjoy, please feel free to leave us a positive review if you like what you are about to read through.

47. KETOGENIC CINNAMON AND CARDAMOM FAT BOMBS

Yield: 10 Servings

Total Time: 45 Minutes

Prep Time: 45 Minutes

Cook Time: 0 Minutes

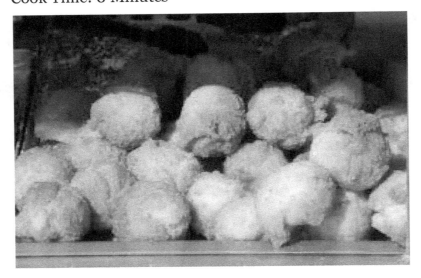

Ingredients:

- 3 oz. butter,
- 5 tablespoons of unsweetened coconut (shredded),
- ½ teaspoon of green ground Cardamom,
- ¼ of a teaspoon of vanilla extract, and
- 1 tablespoon of ground cinnamon.

Directions:

If the butter is not already stored at room temperature, make sure you bring it to the ideal temperature by removing it from the refrigerator. Get a pan, and inside, simply roast the shredded coconut until it becomes brownish a little. Roasting will help create a wonderful flavor, however you can skip this step and simply allow the coconut to cool.

Mix the butter with the half of the shredded coconut alongside the spices, inside the bowl, and then form the mix into Walnut-size balls with the aid of a teaspoon, and roll the remaining shredded coconut inside. Store the mix inside the refrigerator or serve immediately.

Nutritional Information per Serving:

Calories: 341; Total Fat: 31.9 g; Carbs: 5.3 g; Dietary Fiber: 2 g;

Protein: 3.3 g; Cholesterol: 63 mg; Sodium: 147 mg

48. KETO CINNAMON WALNUT POWER MUFFINS

Yield: 12 Servings

Total Time: 40 Minutes

Prep Time: 15 Minutes

Cook Time: 25 Minutes

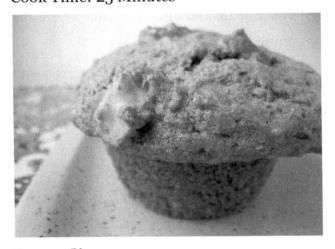

Ingredients:

- 12 ounces of soft cream cheese,
- 5 eggs,
- 2 packets of Splenda (sugar substitute),
- 2 teaspoons of vanilla,
- 1 cup whole almond meal
- 1 cup of unprocessed wheat bran,
- A teaspoon of baking powder,
- 2 teaspoons of ground Cinnamon, and
- A cup chopped of walnuts

Directions:

Pre-heat the oven to 325 degree F and grease 12 muffin pans or cup, or muffin liners. Mix the cream cheese and the eggs in a bowl in an electric mixer. Beat the mix until smooth and other eggs, beat one after the other , and then stir in other ingredients except the walnuts and then stir in the walnuts when other mix have been perfectly blended. Fill in the muffin pans to the brim, and bake for about 25 minutes and serve immediately.

Nutritional Information per Serving:

Calories: 217; Total Fat: 19 g; Carbs: 3 g; Dietary Fiber: 3 g; Protein: 7 g; Cholesterol: 0 mg; Sodium: 0 mg

49. MINI KETOGENIC DONUTS

Yield: 8 Servings

Total Time: 25 Minutes

Prep Time: 15 Minutes

Cook Time: 10 Minutes

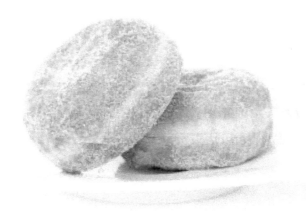

Ingredients:

- 3 oz. of cream cheese,
- 3 medium to large eggs,
- 3 2/3 tablespoons of almond flour,
- 1 ½ tablespoons of coconut flour,
- 1 ½ teaspoons of coconut flour,
- 1 teaspoon of baking powder,
- Teaspoon of vanilla extract,
- 4 teaspoons of erythritol extract, and
- 10 drops of stevia (liquid).

Directions:

With the aid of an immersion blender, gently mix and blend all the ingredients thoroughly, then heat the donut maker up and spray the inside with some coconut oil. Pour the batter equally into the portions of the donut maker. Let the donut batter cook for about 3 minutes on one side and 3 minutes on the other side. Remove the donuts from the donut maker and set the donuts aside to cool and repeat the procedure with the remaining batter if you can't finish them at once.

Nutritional Information per Serving:

Calories: 129; Total Fat: 15 g; Carbs: 5 g; Dietary Fiber: 2 g; Protein: 8 g; Cholesterol: 13 mg; Sodium: 1.1 mg

50. KETOGENIC BLUEBERRY MUFFINS

Yield: 6 Servings

Total Time: 1 Hour

Prep Time: 30 Minutes

Cook Time: 30 Minutes

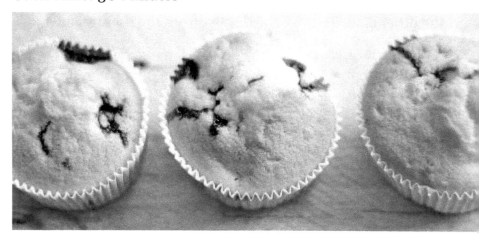

Ingredients:

- 3 large organic eggs,
- ¼ of a cup of a heavy cream or coconut milk,
- 1/3 cup of erythritol crystals,
- 5 tablespoons of organic coconut flour, and
- ½ a cup of frozen organic blueberries.

Directions:

Pre-heat your oven to about 350-degree F, and line your muffin pans with some paper liners. Get a large bowl and inside, whisk the egg with the erythritol and cream before mixing very well. Add your coconut flour to the egg mix and whisk the mixture until it becomes smooth. Wait for the mix to settle for about 5 minutes until the batter becomes thickened. Add your frozen blueberries, and mix further. Let the batter settle for about 2 minutes and then scoop it inside the muffin cups. Bake the muffins for about 30 minutes until you are able to insert a stick or fork in the middle of the muffins and it comes out clean. Let the muffins cool before serving.

Nutritional Information per Serving:

Calories: 217; Total Fat: 19 g; Carbs: 3 g; Dietary Fiber: 3 g; Protein: 7 g; Cholesterol: 0 mg; Sodium: 0 mg

51. LOW CARB CINNAMON DONUTS

Yield: 8 Servings

Total Time: 1 Hour

Prep Time: 45 Minutes

Cook Time: 15 Minutes

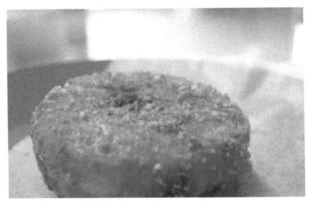

Ingredients:

For the donut, you need the following ingredients;

- 1 cup of almond flour,
- ¼ of a cup of granulated erythritol,
- 2 tablespoons of vanilla protein powder,
- Teaspoon of cinnamon (ground),
- 1 teaspoon of baking powder,
- ¼ teaspoon of sea salt
- 3 tablespoons of melted butter ,
- 2lightly beaten eggs,
- ¼ of a cup of almond milk,
- 8-10 drops of liquid stevia (sugar alternative),
- ¼ of a teaspoon of vanilla extract.

For the Glaze, you need the following ingredients;

- 3 teaspoons of butter,
- 6 tablespoons of erythritol (powdered),
- 2 tablespoons of heavy cream, and
- ¼ of a teaspoon of vanilla extract.

Directions:

To make the donuts, simply grease the donut pan, and then pre-heat the oven to about 350-degree F. Get a large bowl and inside whisk together the erythritol, almond flour, cinnamon, protein powder, salt and baking powder. Inside the bowl, gently stir in the melted butter alongside the eggs, stevia, almond milk, and vanilla extract until they are well combined.

Fill the donut pan with until each hole is about 2/3 full and then bake them for about 17 minutes until the donuts are light brown in color, and make sure they are set. Let the donuts cool for about 5 minutes inside the pan and after baking, before flipping them into a wire rack and then cool further for about 5 minutes. Repeat this baking with the remaining donut batter.

To make the glaze, melt your butter inside the small skillet and over medium heat. Make sure the butter is cooked until it becomes brown and fragrant, this should take around 4 minutes, then remove from heat. Get a medium bowl and inside, place the erythritol, then whisk in the browned butter until the mixture becomes thick and perfectly combined. Stir in the cream (1 tablespoon at a time), until you are able to achieve a spreadable consistency. Stir in your vanilla extract, and then spread the glaze on top of the donut, and let the glaze set for about 20 minutes before serving.

Nutritional Information per Serving:

Calories: 141; Total Fat: 12 g; Carbs: 2 g; Dietary Fiber: 0 g; Protein: 4 g; Cholesterol: 0 mg; Sodium: 0 mg

52. LOW CARB PEANUT BUTTER CHOCOLATE CHIP MUFFINS

Yield: 6 Servings

Total Time: 40 Minutes

Prep Time: 25 Minutes

Cook Time: 15 Minutes

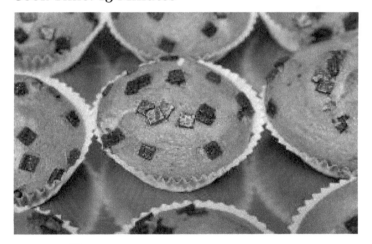

Ingredients:

- ½ a cup of almond flour,
- ½ a cup of erythritol,
- 1 tablespoon of baking powder,
- ½ a teaspoon of salt,
- 1/3 of a cup of peanut butter,
- 1/3 of a cup of almond milk,
- 2 moderate to large eggs,
- ½ a cup of cacao nips (or zero-sugar chocolate chips).

Directions:

Pre-heat the oven to 350-degree F, and then get a mixing bowl where you combine all the dry ingredients and stir properly. Add your peanut butter into the mix, and then add almond milk before your stir to combine further. Add an egg at a time, and stir until each egg has been fully combined. Fold in your cacao nibs or zero-sugar chocolate chips, then spray your muffin tin with a cooking spray and then distribute the batter evenly to make 6 large muffins. Bake the muffins for about 15 minutes, and cool them off then add some butter or zero sugar maple syrup.

Nutritional Information per Serving:

Calories: 174; Total Fat: 16.9 g; Carbs: 1.2 g; Dietary Fiber: 0 g;

Protein: 6.9 g; Cholesterol: 0 mg; Sodium: 0 mg

Conclusion

You did it! Congrats on getting all the way to the end of our Keto Bread Cookbook: For Keto, Paleo & Gluten free Diets! This was indeed your very first hurdle to becoming a master of creating Keto Breads, and the first of many positive hurdles to come as you travel along this Keto road.

I hope you have enjoyed all 52 delicious Keto bread recipes, and that you will continue to enjoy them with your whole family.

What happens next?

The next step is to continue practicing and enjoying the recipes as you see fit. Then when you are ready to begin another adventure join us again on yet another one of our amazing culinary journeys. Remember to leave us a positive review if you liked what you read.

Until next time, keep on cooking. Best of luck!

CPSIA information can be obtained
at www.ICGtesting.com
Printed in the USA
BVHW040627151120
593358BV00014B/273